Reading Medical English in the News

ニュースで読む
医療英語

CD付き

川越栄子〈編著〉

森 茂・田中芳文
名木田恵理子・大下晴美〈著〉

講談社

執筆者一覧

編著者

川越栄子　　　滋慶医療科学大学　教授（1, 9, 10）

著者

森　茂　　　　大分大学　教授（2, 5, 7）

田中芳文　　　島根県立大学　教授（4, 6, 15）

名木田恵理子　元川崎医療短期大学　教授（8, 11, 12）

大下晴美　　　大分大学　准教授（3, 13, 14）

（　）内は執筆担当章

まえがき

　超高齢化社会を迎えた日本において、「医療」は国民の最大の関心事となっています。日本は医療レベルが高く、医療保険制度も世界一との評価を得ています。研究においてもiPS細胞など世界のトップレベルの医学研究を行っている分野も数多くあります。一方、高齢者介護、医師不足、医療事故、心の病など抱えている課題も多いです。

　世界に目を向けると、諸外国の多くは日本とは異なる医療文化を持ち、医師を育てる教育においても違ったシステムを持っています。また、現在でも水や衛生上の問題などで病を発症し幼児死亡率の高い国々も存在しています。

　このような国内外の医療問題について英語ニュースを通して知っていただくというのが本書の大きな目的です。The Japan Times, Voice of America, The Daily Yomiuriに取り上げられた医療ニュースを厳選し、大学医学科・看護学科の学生に長年医療英語の講義をしている著者が、医療のさまざまなテーマについて解説をし、英語学習のための問題・英語文法を執筆いたしました。医療系学部学生、医療関係者はもとより、広くさまざまな分野の方に読んでいただきたいと考えています。

　本書は、「日常の健康」「多い病気」「医療の形」「医療にまつわる問題」「世界の医療」の5本の柱を建て、それぞれのトピックに対して興味深い記事を選びました。万人にとって大切な「日常の健康」を保つための病気予防法を知っていただき、日本人に「多い病気」である癌・うつ病、世界に多いエイズについて学んでいただきます。さらにさまざまな「医療の形」（救急医療、災害医療、代替医療、高度医療等）について知識を得ていただきます。そして、現在のネット社会、高齢出産増加、医療のグローバル化に伴う「医療にまつわる問題」について考えていただきます。最後に日本とは異なる「世界の医療」についての例を読んでいただくという構成になっています。目次に見られるように、タイトルでどのようなトピックであるかを示しましたので、読者の興味あるトピックから読み進めていただければ結構です。なお、CDも付けていますので、英文を聴くことでさらに内容の理解を深めると共に、医療英語の発音も確認していただきたいと思います。

　このように幅広く日本・世界の医療について知識を得て理解を深めていただくと共に、英語読解力も高められるように工夫しています。英語力の高い読者は、(Vocabulary Check)で用語を

まず確認してから、時間を計ってできるだけ速く読んでください。英文の後にwpm（1分間で読める語彙数）を出せるようになっていますのでご自分のwpmを把握してください。英語のネイテイブスピーカーであれば1分間に約300語のスピードで英語を読めます。英語ニュースは1分間約200語で話されているといわれています。日本の大学生が1分間に読むことができる英語は100語以下の場合が多いです。wpmを上げるためには「習うより慣れろ！」です。概要を把握しながらできるだけ速く読む練習をして、まずは、1分間150語をめざしてください。さらに、英文を読まずに内容把握問題を解き正確に理解できているかを確認してください。巻末にある解答で採点し、正解率をwpmの値にかけて読解効率を算出し、各回記録して速読力を上げる努力をしてください。英語力に自信のない方は、各自のペースで一語一語時間をかけてゆっくりと精読してください。英文読解後、語句問題を解き重要語句を確認してください。

また、各章文法の重要事項について解説しています。英語から長年離れていた読者も英文法の基本を復習することで、英語学習を再開していただきたいと思います。文法解説の例文・文法問題は出来る限り医療用語を使い、自然に医療英語に慣れていただくよう工夫しました。

さらに、各章の最後に「Let's think」「Let's make a speech]「コラム」を入れ、各トピックについて読者の考えを発展させていただき、スピーチ・デイスカッションの練習もできるようにしています。日本人は英語でのスピーチ・デイスカッションの経験がない人が多いですが、このような技能は「グローバリゼーション」が進むなかで、今までよりもさらに重要になってくることは確実です。英語が苦手であれば、最初は日本語から始めて英語に切り替えていくというようなやり方をとられるのも良いと思います。

上記のように、本書は、医療のプロフェッショナルだけでなく、医療に関心を持つ幅広い読者層を対象にしています。各読者の英語力に合わせて、速読・精読どちらでも対応できるようにしています。英語を基礎から学びたい人のためには基本英文法も解説しています。また、読解力をあげるのみならず、スピーチ・デイスカッションもできるようにも工夫しています。

さまざまな読者層が、レベル・必要に応じて英語で医療について学び活用できるようにしたのが本書の特徴です。個々人に合ったさまざまな方法で本書を活用していただければ幸いです。

2014年8月

編著者

Contents

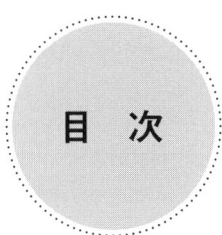

目次

まえがき iii

日常の健康

Chapter 1 賢く飲み、賢く食べて、健やかに

A. Green Tea, Coffee May Cut Stroke Risk CD Track 01 1

B. Moderation Best for Eating Meat, Milk Products CD Track 02 3

  文法解説【文型】 5

  Column　食事をバランスよく摂り健康に！ 7

Chapter 2 風邪って何だろう？

What Do You Know about the Common Cold? CD Track 03 10

  文法解説【文の種類】 13

  Column　風邪（感冒）（common cold）とインフルエンザ（influenza） ... 15

多い病気

Chapter 3 がん撲滅への道

WHO: One-Third of All Cancer Deaths Are Preventable CD Track 04 ... 16

  文法解説【関係代名詞】 19

  Column　がん 22

Chapter 4　日本人気質もうつ病の原因?

Depression Is a National Ailment That Demands Open Recognition in Japan　CD Track 05 …… 24

文法解説【関係副詞】……… 27

Column　緊急救命室での精神疾患 ……… 29

Chapter 5　エイズ対策は国際的規模で

Eight Million People Now Being Treated for HIV　CD Track 06 …… 30

文法解説【分詞構文】……… 33

Column　世界エイズデーとレッドリボン ……… 35

医療の形

Chapter 6　「救急ヘリ」と「救急車」どちらを選ぶ?

Medevac Copters Soon to Cover Entire Nation　CD Track 07 …… 36

文法解説【分詞】……… 39

Column　日本のドクターヘリはこれから? ……… 41

Chapter 7　ハンズオンリーCPRであなたも人命が救えます

Hands-Only CPR Is a Simpler Way to Save Lives　CD Track 08 …… 42

文法解説【不定詞】……… 45

Column　CPRのA-B-C ……… 47

Chapter 8　災害医療には心のケアも並行して

Mental Health Must Match Post-3/11 Recovery　CD Track 09 …… 48

文法解説【動名詞】……… 51

Column　大災害の後は継続的な心身のケア体制が必要 ……… 53

Chapter 9 : 笑いは最高の妙薬

India's Giggling Guru Counsels Laughing Yourself to Good Health （CD Track 10） …… 54

- 文法解説【受動態】 …… 57
- Column❶ 「統合医療」（Integrative Medicine） …… 59
- Column❷ 映画 *Patch Adams* …… 59

Chapter 10 : iPSは人類の夢

World's First Clinical Trials with Human iPS Cells OK'd （CD Track 11） …… 60

- 文法解説【仮定法】 …… 63
- Column iPS 細胞 …… 65

医療にまつわる問題

Chapter 11 : 薬のネット販売に一定のルールを

Rules for Online Drug Sales （CD Track 12） …… 66

- 文法解説【疑問詞】 …… 69
- Column 薬のインターネット販売が解禁されるまで …… 71

Chapter 12 : 血液検査による出生前診断、始まる

New Prenatal Diagnosis May Start Next Month （CD Track 13） …… 72

- 文法解説【否定形】 …… 75
- Column 新型出生前診断：命にかかわる重い検査 …… 77

Chapter 13 : 医療通訳で大切なことは？

The Risks of Language for Health Translators （CD Track 14） …… 78

- 文法解説【命令文】 …… 81
- Column 医療ツーリズムと医療通訳 …… 83

世界の医療

Chapter 14 : 世界の子どもたちの現状を知ろう！

Fewer Children under Age 5 Are Dying (CD Track 15) 84

- 文法解説【時制】........ 87
- **Column** ミレニアム開発目標（Millennium Development Goals：MDGs）........ 89

Chapter 15 : 医師になるのはいばらの道

So You Want to Make Your Mother Happy? Become a Doctor (CD Track 16) 90

- 文法解説【品詞】........ 93
- **Column** 「アメリカの医学教育」........ 95

解答 97

本文イラスト：北原志乃

Chapter 1　賢く飲み、賢く食べて、健やかに

「医食同源」とは、バランスの取れた食事をとることで病気を予防・治療しようとする考え方です。緑茶・コーヒーの効用、肉・乳製品の食べ方についての記事を読んで、自分の食生活を見直してみましょう。

CD Track 01

A.　Green Tea, Coffee May Cut Stroke Risk

Vocabulary Check（英文を読む前に意味を確認しましょう。）

- stroke：脳卒中　 ● blood vessel：血管　 ● National Cancer Center：国立がん研究センター
- National Cerebral and Cardiovascular Center：国立循環器病研究センター
- health center：医療センター　 ● jurisdiction：管轄　 ● brain hemorrhage：脳出血
- subarachnoid bleeding：くも膜下出血　 ● abstain from ～：～を控える

・自信のある人は英文をできるだけ速く読み、時間を計ってください。苦手な人はゆっくり読みましょう。

　A study tracking more than 80,000 adults for 13 years found those who regularly drank green tea or coffee were 20 percent less likely to suffer a stroke, researchers said on Friday. Green tea may help protect blood vessels, while coffee could lower blood sugar levels, according to the study by the National Cancer Center in Tokyo and the National Cerebral and Cardiovascular Center in Osaka.

　The team followed some 82,000 people aged between 45 and 74 in nine public health center jurisdictions in the late 1990s. In the tracking period, 3,425 people suffered various forms of stroke, such as brain hemorrhage and subarachnoid bleeding. Compared with those who abstained from green tea or coffee, those who drank at least one cup of green tea each day had a 22 to 35 percent lower risk of suffering a brain hemorrhage. The risk of a stroke was 14 to 20 percent lower among those who drank two to three cups daily, the study found. For coffee, those who drank three to six cups a week had an 11 to 20 percent lower risk of experiencing a stroke.

(185 words)

(The Japan Times, Mar. 16, 2013)

(共同通信配信)

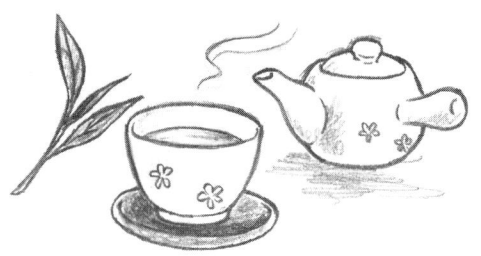
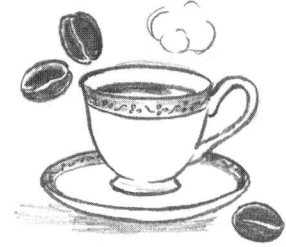

速読をした人はwpmを確認しましょう。前ページの英文を2分で読めた人のwpmは93になります。

計算式：（あなたのwpm）＝ 総単語数（185）/（かかった時間（分））　　　　あなたのwpm：　　　　　wpm

（参考）　45秒　247wpm　　　1分　185wpm　　　1.5分　123wpm
　　　　　2分　93wpm　　　2.5分　74wpm

wpmとはwords per minute（一分間に読める語彙数）のことです。英語のネイテイブスピーカーであれば1分間に約300語のスピードで英語を読めます。一方、日本の大学生が1分間に読むことができる英語は100語以下の場合が多いといわれています。wpmを上げるためには、「習うより慣れろ！」です。多くの英文を、訳するのではなく、概要を把握しながら、できるだけ速く読む練習をしてください。まずは、1分間150語をめざしてください。（TOEICのリーデイングパートをすべて解くのに必要な速度は1分間に150語といわれています。）

内容把握問題　次の1～5の英文が、本文の内容と一致する場合はT、一致しない場合はFを（　）内に記入しましょう。

1. (　) People who drink green tea or coffee are less likely to suffer strokes.
2. (　) Drinking green tea lowers blood sugar levels.
3. (　) Drinking coffee may lower blood sugar levels.
4. (　) The study was done in nine health center jurisdictions.
5. (　) People who drink two cups of coffee a week have lower risk of experiencing strokes.

上記の問題はいくつできましたか？　正解率をあなたのwpmの値にかけてみましょう。

計算式：（あなたの読解効率）＝（あなたのwpm）×（（正答数）/ 5）　　　　あなたの読解効率：

速く、かつ正確に読むことが求められます。

語句問題　本文中に出てくる次の1～5の語句とほぼ同じ意味を表すものをa～dの中から1つ選びましょう。

1. track
　　a. run　　　　　　b. follow　　　　　c. interview　　　　d. find
2. regularly
　　a. seldom　　　　b. often　　　　　　c. rarely　　　　　　d. weekly
3. suffer
　　a. avoid　　　　　b. hit　　　　　　　c. decrease　　　　　d. experience
4. various
　　a. different　　　　b. difficult　　　　 c. same　　　　　　 d. few
5. abstain
　　a. contain　　　　b. sustain　　　　　c. obtain　　　　　　d. refrain

B. Moderation Best for Eating Meat, Milk Products

Vocabulary Check （英文を読む前に意味を確認しましょう。）

- consume：消費する、過度に食べる　- saturated fatty acids：飽和脂肪酸
- dairy product：乳製品　- heart attack：心臓発作　- moderately：適度に
- in accordance with ～：～に従って　- body：機関　- classify：分類する　- subject：対象者
- intake：摂取　- incidence：発生率　- ingest：摂取する　- cholesterol：コレステロール

・自信のある人は英文をできるだけ速く読み、時間を計ってください。苦手な人はゆっくり読みましょう。

People who consume a lot of saturated fatty acids contained in meat and dairy products are less likely to be hit by stroke but face a larger risk of heart attack, a recent study by the National Cancer Center and other bodies found. "It is good to eat meat and milk products moderately," the center said, based on a study of around 82,000 people in Japan.

They classified the subjects into five groups in accordance with their intakes, and found that the incidence of strokes among those who take in the largest amount of fatty acids at 21.6-96.7 grams a day is 23 percent lower than among those who ingest the smallest amount at 0.8-11.7 grams per day. Intake of saturated fatty acid is believed to increase cholesterol that strengthens blood vessels.

In contrast, the incidence of heart attacks among the biggest consumers of fatty acids is 39 percent higher than among those who eat the least amount. Thus taking in some 20 grams of saturated fatty acid, equivalent to 200 grams of milk a day, and 150 grams of meat every other day, is considered a safe diet.

（190 words）
（The Japan Times, Mar. 15, 2013）
（共同通信配信）

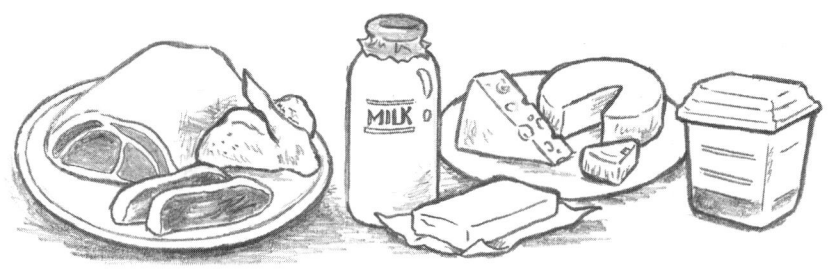

速読をした人は wpm を確認しましょう。

計算式：（あなたの wpm）＝総単語数(190) / （かかった時間(分)）　　あなたの wpm：　　　　　wpm

（参考）　45秒　253wpm　　　　1分　190wpm　　　　1.5分　127wpm
　　　　　2分　95wpm　　　　2.5分　76wpm

内容把握問題　次の 1 〜 5 の英文が、本文の内容と一致する場合は T、一致しない場合は F を（ ）内に記入しましょう。

1. (　　) The subjects were divided into two groups.
2. (　　) People who consume a lot of saturated fatty acids, such as those contained in meat and dairy products are more likely to have strokes.
3. (　　) The National Cancer Center classified the people according to age.
4. (　　) Moderate consumption of saturated fatty acids is healthy.
5. (　　) The incidence of heart attacks among the smallest consumers of fatty acids is very high.

上記の問題はいくつできましたか？　正解率をあなたの wpm の値にかけてみましょう。

計算式：（あなたの読解効率）＝（あなたの wpm）×（(正答数)/5）　　あなたの読解効率：

語句問題　本文中に出てくる次の 1 〜 5 の語句とほぼ同じ意味を表すものを a 〜 d の中から 1 つ選びましょう。

1. consume
    a. discard　　　b. eat　　　c. make　　　d. change
2. contain
    a. exclude　　　b. include　　　c. maintain　　　d. digest
3. around
    a. more than　　　b. probably　　　c. exactly　　　d. about
4. equivalent
    a. different　　　b. small　　　c. approximate　　　d. equal
5. diet
    a. fat　　　b. weight　　　c. food　　　d. drink

文法解説【文型】

英語の文は原則として、主語、動詞、目的語、補語、修飾語から構成されています。これをもとに文を分類すると、基本的には次の 5 つの型になります。

第 1 文型　S ＋ V（主語＋動詞）「S が（は）…する」
　【例】The man is bleeding.
　※第 1 文型に使われる動詞：live, cough, walk, laugh, sleep, etc.

第 2 文型　S ＋ V ＋ C（主語＋動詞＋補語）「S は C である（になる）」
　【例（本文）】The risk of stroke was 14 to 20 percent lower.
　※第 2 文型に使われる動詞：be 動詞 , become, keep, seem, look, appear, fall, feel, remain, turn, etc.

第 3 文型　S ＋ V ＋ O（主語＋動詞＋目的語）「S は O を…する」
　【例（本文）】The team followed some 82,000 people.
　※第 3 文型に使われる動詞：have, want, help, decide, eat, like, take, put, finish, borrow, enjoy, etc.

第 4 文型　S ＋ V ＋ O_1 ＋ O_2（主語＋動詞＋目的語 $_1$ ＋目的語 $_2$）「S は O_1 に O_2 を…する」
　【例】The nurse showed the patient the way to the elevator.
　※第 4 文型に使われる動詞：give, lend, tell, pass, buy, make, send, ask, promise, etc.

第 5 文型　S ＋ V ＋ O ＋ C（主語＋動詞＋目的語＋補語）「S は O を C にする／O を C と思う」など
　【例】The patient found the doctor great.
　※第 5 文型に使われる動詞：call, name, find, elect, leave, make, etc.

文法問題　次の 1 〜 10 の英文が、第 1 〜 5 文型のどれか答えましょう。

1. My friend had surgery last month.　　　　　　　　　　　　　第（　　）文型
2. The doctor left the patient alone.　　　　　　　　　　　　　第（　　）文型
3. Please walk slowly.　　　　　　　　　　　　　　　　　　　第（　　）文型
4. The patient is sleeping now.　　　　　　　　　　　　　　　第（　　）文型
5. My mother regularly drinks green tea.　　　　　　　　　　　第（　　）文型
6. The doctor gave me some advice.　　　　　　　　　　　　　第（　　）文型
7. It is good to moderately consume meat and milk products.　　第（　　）文型
8. Coffee made me more awake.　　　　　　　　　　　　　　　第（　　）文型
9. Coffee might lower blood sugar levels.　　　　　　　　　　　第（　　）文型
10. Moderately consuming saturated fatty acids is necessary for good health.　第（　　）文型

英作文　次の1～5の日本文を（　）内の指示に従って英語になおしましょう。

1. その患者さんは松葉杖（crutches）なしで歩くことができない。（第1文型を使って）
2. 今日は調子（気分）がよい。（第2文型でfeelを使って）
3. 胃（おなか）が痛い。（第3文型を使って）
4. 彼は私に杖（walking stick）を貸してくれた。（第4文型を使って）
5. 私は主治医が誠実だとわかった。（第5文型を使って）

Let's think!

あなたの昨日の食事を思い出して、食材名を英語で書きだしてみましょう。（【例】egg, milk, rice）そして、後述のコラムで紹介する「食事バランスガイド」にあてはめてみて、適切な食事ができているかどうか検証してみましょう。

Let's make a speech!

健康を保つための食生活について、参考文献やインターネットなどを調べてまとめ、英語で3分間のスピーチをしてみましょう。

> **Column**
> [コラム]
>
> ## 食事をバランスよく摂り健康に！

厚生労働省と農林水産省から「食事バランスガイド」が出されています。
コマのイラストにより、一日分の食事を表現し、これらの食事のバランスが悪いと倒れてしまうことを表現しています。あなたのコマはうまくまわっているでしょうか？

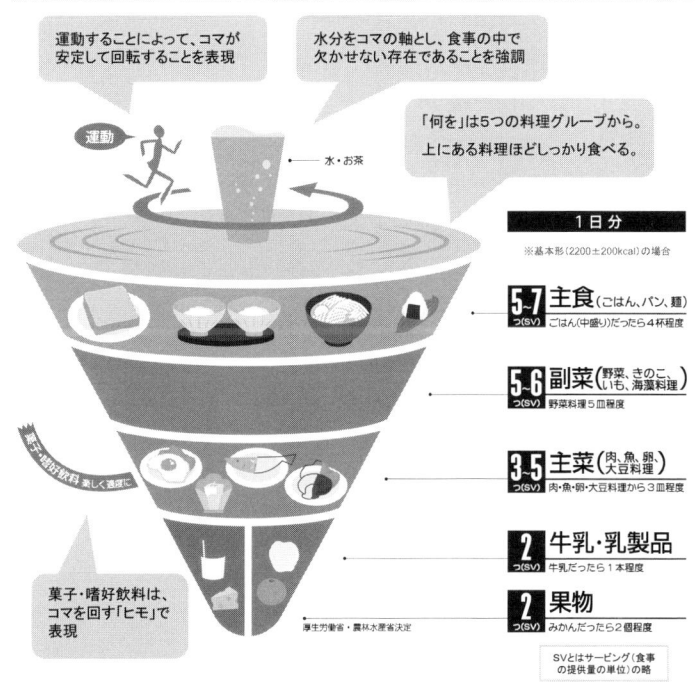

●食事の適量（どれだけ食べたらよいか）は、性別、年齢、活動量によって異なります。コマのイラストは2200±200kcal（基本形）の場合の目安です。
●自分の適量を確認し、毎日の食事をチェックしてみましょう。

あなたの適量を調べてみましょう。
（農林水産省ホームページ）
http://www.maff.go.jp/j/balance_guide/

check! まずは、自分の一日分の適量を調べましょう

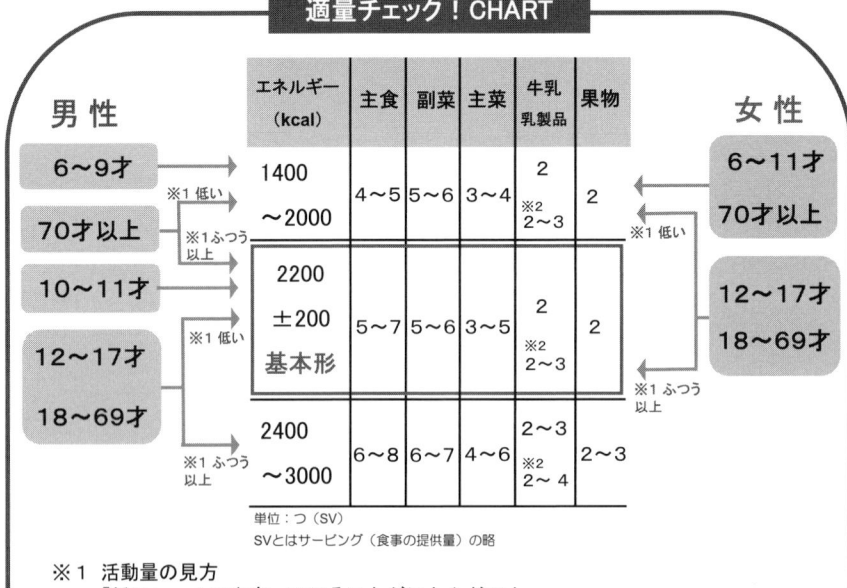

※1 活動量の見方
「低い」：1日中座っていることがほとんどの人
「ふつう以上」：「低い」に該当しない人

さらに強い運動や労働を行っている人は、適宜調整が必要です。

※2 学校給食を含めた子ども向け摂取目安について
成長期に特に必要なカルシウムを十分にとるためにも、牛乳・乳製品の適量は少し幅を持たせて1日2～3つ（SV）、「基本形」よりもエネルギー量が多い場合では、4つ（SV）程度までを目安にするのが適当です。

check! 自分の1日の適量を、書き込みましょう。

エネルギー	主食	副菜	主菜	牛乳・乳製品	果物
kcal	つ（SV）	つ（SV）	つ（SV）	つ（SV）	つ（SV）

Chapter 2　風邪って何だろう？

あなたは「風邪（common cold）」についてどれくらい知っていますか？
風邪は寒いとひくのでしょうか？　またどのようにして伝染するのでしょうか？　そして治療法は？

CD Track 03

What Do You Know about the Common Cold?

Vocabulary Check（英文を読む前に意味を確認しましょう。）

- cure：治す、治療法
- temperature：温度、気温
- congregate：集まる
- virus：ウイルス
- transmit：伝染させる
- handshake：握手
- sneeze：くしゃみをする
- cough：咳をする
- resistant：耐性のある
- infect：感染させる
- immunity：免疫（性）
- symptom：症状
- duration：存続期間
- the Agriculture Department：（米国）農務省
- prepared food：加工〔調理された〕食品
- treat：処置する、手当てする
- anti-inflammatory：抗炎症性の
- mucus：粘液
- sticky：粘着性のある
- breathe：呼吸する
- saying：言い習わし
- starve：飢えさせる
- fever：発熱
- fluid：液体
- secretion：分泌（物）
- thicken：濃くする
- discomfort：不快感

・自信のある人は英文をできるだけ速く読み、時間を計ってください。苦手な人はゆっくり読みましょう。

　　Do you think getting cold can give you a cold? Is it bad to drink milk when you have a cold? Can chicken soup cure a cold?

　　Ranit Mishori is a family medicine doctor at Georgetown University Medical Center in Washington. She says colds are more common in winter, but not because of low temperatures. The cold weather just means people stay inside more. "People tend to congregate and be together and the way the common cold virus is transmitted from one person to another is through handshakes, through sneezing, or coughing on one another."

　　Adults generally get two to three colds a year. Children are likely to catch four or five. Dr. Mishori says some people mistakenly believe they can become resistant to colds. "There are about two hundred different viruses that cause the common cold. People think that once you get infected one time you develop immunity for the rest of your life. This is wrong."

　　There is still no cure for the common cold. But Dr. Mishori says there are ways to feel better sooner. "So if you get a cold and on day one and you start taking about two grams of vitamin C a day, there is evidence that it might shorten the number of days that you will be suffering with these symptoms."

　　She says honey can also help. "There is increased evidence that it helps shorten the duration of the common cold sometimes even by two to three days." Dr. Mishori says honey seems to be especially effective in children with colds. But the Agriculture

Department says never to feed honey to babies less than one year old. It says even honey in prepared foods may contain substances that can make babies very sick.

　Some people believe in treating a cold with chicken soup. Does it work? "Chicken soup has anti-inflammatory properties, so it helps reduce the duration of the cold but also it helps clear the mucus." Mucus is the sticky substance that can make you cough and have trouble breathing during a cold.

　Have you ever heard the old saying "feed a cold, starve a fever"? Dr. Mishori says this is not necessarily a good guideline to follow. She says if you have a cold but do not feel hungry, then don't eat. "But you have to drink a lot and you can drink water or you can drink tea — anything that gets fluids into your body. That's very important."

　But what about drinking milk during a cold? Some people think it only causes more mucus. Dr. Mishori says yes and no. "Dairy products do not cause increased secretions, but they can thicken the secretions. So it's possible that discomfort is somewhat more enhanced when you drink milk. But obviously, if you're a baby and that's all you drink, you should not stop giving babies milk."

(476 words)

(Voice of America, Apr. 20, 2011)

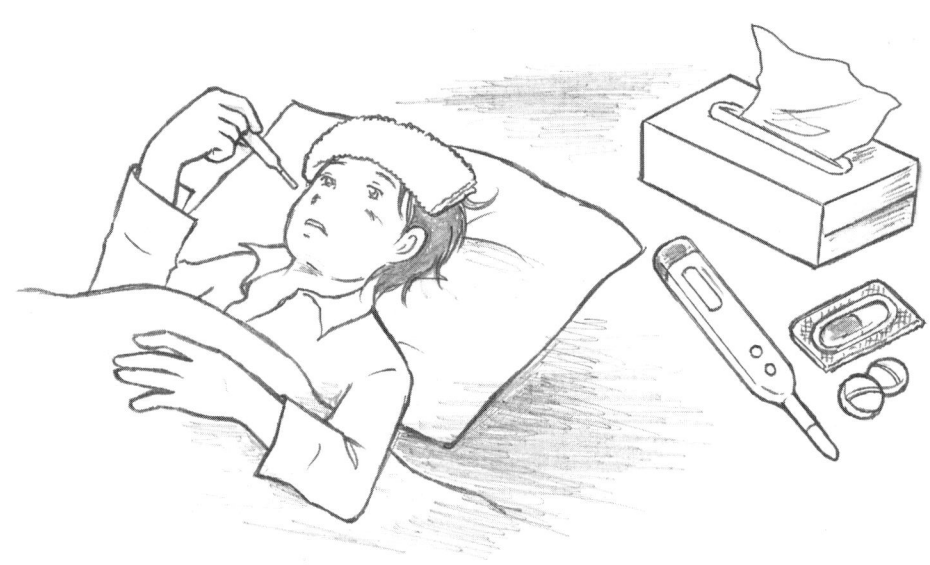

速読をした人は wpm を確認しましょう。

計算式：（あなたの wpm）＝総単語数(476)／（かかった時間(分)）　　　**あなたの wpm：　　　　wpm**

（参考）
2分	238wpm	2.5分	190wpm	3分	159wpm
3.5分	136wpm	4分	119wpm	4.5分	106wpm
5分	95wpm	5.5分	87wpm	6分	79wpm

内容把握問題　次の1〜5の英文が、本文の内容と一致する場合は T、一致しない場合は F を（ ）内に記入しましょう。

1. (　) Common colds are more prevalent in winter because temperatures are low.
2. (　) Once you are infected with common cold viruses, you become immune for the rest of your life.
3. (　) The old saying "feed a cold, starve a fever" means you should eat when you feel cold and not eat when you have a fever.
4. (　) It is very important to get a lot of fluids when you have a cold.
5. (　) If you drink milk while you have a cold, you may feel uncomfortable.

上記の問題はいくつできましたか？　正解率をあなたの wpm の値にかけてみましょう。

計算式：（あなたの読解効率）＝（あなたの wpm）×（（正答数）／ 5）　　　**あなたの読解効率：**

語句問題　本文中に出てくる次の1〜5の語句とほぼ同じ意味を表すものを a 〜 d の中から1つ選びましょう。

1. evidence
    a. proof　　　b. document　　　c. display　　　d. statement
2. substance
    a. gas　　　b. matter　　　c. volume　　　d. poison
3. property
    a. accuracy　　　b. characteristic　　　c. politeness　　　d. function
4. enhance
    a. encourage　　　b. relieve　　　c. increase　　　d. transfer
5. reduce
    a. make something better　　　b. make something worse
    c. make something more　　　d. make something less

文法解説【文の種類】

☆ 文（sentence）は構造的な視点からみると、次の3種類に分類されます。

① **単文** 主語（S）が1つ、動詞（V）が1つで構成されているもの
【例（本文）】Adults generally get two to three colds a year.

② **重文** 単文が等位接続詞（and, but, or, for, so, nor, yet）で結ばれているもの
【例（本文）】Dairy products do not cause increased secretions, but they can thicken secretions.

③ **複文** 単文が従属接続詞（等位接続詞以外の接続詞や関係詞）で結ばれているもの
【例（本文）】She says (that) colds are more common in winter.

☆ 文を内容の点からみると、次の4種類に分類されます。

① **平叙文** 何かを伝える文で、通常 S + V + 〜の形をとり、終止符（．）で終わります。
【例（本文）】The cold weather just means people stay inside more.

② **疑問文** 何かを尋ねる文で、疑問符（？）で終わります。
疑問文には、一般疑問文（Yes / No で答える疑問文）、選択疑問文（or を用いる疑問文）、特殊疑問文（疑問詞を用いる疑問文）があります。
【例（本文）】Do you think getting cold can give you a cold?

③ **命令文** 何かを命令・依頼する文で、通例主語 You を省略し動詞の原形で始まります。
【例】Speak English in this class.
Do not take this medicine with tea.

④ **感嘆文** 喜びや驚きなどの気持ちを表す文で、次の形式をとり、感嘆符（！）で終わります。
① How + 形容詞 / 副詞 + S + V 〜！
② What a〔an〕+ 形容詞 + 名詞 + S + V 〜！
【例】What a good speaker of English you are!

文法問題

A 次の1～5の文が単文、重文、複文のどれか答えましょう。
1. Ranit Mishori is a family doctor. (　　　)
2. Chicken soup has anti-inflammatory properties, which helps reduce the duration of a cold. (　　　)
3. I wanted to go to school, but my doctor told me to stay in bed. (　　　)
4. Children are likely to catch four or five colds a year. (　　　)
5. When you have a cold, you may have a high fever, a runny nose, and a cough. (　　　)

B 日本語を参考に、次の1～5の英文の（　）内に適語を入れましょう。
1. 糖尿病は、体が十分なインスリンを生成しない場合に発症します。
   Diabetes occurs when your body (　　　)(　　　)(　　　) enough insulin.
2. あなたは病院で生まれましたか、それとも家で生まれましたか。
   (　　　) you born in the hospital, (　　　) at home?
3. どのくらい入院しなければなりませんか。
   (　　　)(　　　)(　　　) I (　　　) to stay in the hospital?
4. 1歳未満の赤ちゃんにはちみつを与えてはいけません。
   (　　　) feed honey to babies less than one year of age.
5. なんて顔色が悪いんでしょう。
   (　　　) pale you look!

英作文 次の1～5の日本文を（　）内の指示に従って英語になおしましょう。
1. 咳がひどいです。（平叙文で）
2. 食欲（appetite）はどうですか。（疑問詞を用いた疑問文で）
3. 熱があるときは、この薬を飲んでください。（命令文で）
4. 食事（meal）の前に手を洗いましたか。（Yes / No で答える疑問文で）
5. 風邪をひいている時には、鼻をかむ（blow one's nose）ことが大切です。（平叙文で）

Let's think!

「風邪は万病のもと」（A cold often leads to all kinds of disease.）といわれるように風邪を甘くみていてはいけません。風邪をひかない予防策としてどのようなことが考えられますか？　英語で説明してみましょう。

Let's make a speech!

風邪をひいたときの症状・治療法について、参考文献やインターネットなどを調べてまとめ、英語で3分スピーチをしてみましょう。

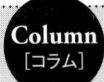

風邪（感冒）(common cold) とインフルエンザ(influenza)

　風邪とインフルエンザは似たような症状がみられますが、一般的に風邪のほうが症状がより軽く（milder）、肺炎（pneumonia）など重症化することは少ないです。おもな症状の違いは以下の通りです。

風邪：鼻水（ruuny nose）、鼻詰まり（stuffy nose）、咽頭痛（のどの痛み）(sore throat)、
　　　くしゃみ（sneezing）、咳（coughing）

インフルエンザ：高熱 (high fever)、体の痛み（body aches）、
　　　　　　　　極度の疲労（extreme tiredness）、空咳（痰などが出ない咳 dry cough）

以下のサイトで確認しましょう。
http://www.cdc.gov/getsmart/antibiotic-use/URI/colds.html
http://www.cdc.gov/flu/about/qa/coldflu.htm

Chapter 3　がん撲滅への道

厚生労働省の平成24年人口動態統計月報年計によると、日本人の死因順位は1位 悪性新生物（がん）、2位 心疾患、3位 肺炎となっています。がん対策の現状に関するWHOの調査概要を読んで、がん予防について考えてみましょう。

CD Track 04

WHO: One-Third of All Cancer Deaths Are Preventable

Vocabulary Check（英文を読む前に意味を確認しましょう。）

- World Health Organization (WHO)：世界保健機関　● World Cancer Day：世界対がんデー
- diagnose：診断する
- Department for Chronic Diseases and Health Promotion：慢性疾患と健康増進部門
- outlook：将来の展望　● grim：厳しい　● physical inactivity：運動不足　● obesity：肥満
- metropolitan：大都市（の）　● stave off：～を防ぐ　● vaccination：ワクチン接種
- infection：感染症　● hepatitis B：B型肝炎　● vaccinate：ワクチン接種をする
- human papilloma virus：ヒト乳頭腫ウイルス　● cervical cancer：子宮頸がん
- vaccine：ワクチン　● screen：検査する　● implementation：実施

・自信のある人は英文をできるだけ速く読み、時間を計ってください。苦手な人はゆっくり読みましょう。

　The World Health Organization reports one-third of all cancer deaths are preventable. But, a global survey prepared for World Cancer Day, Monday, finds more than half of all countries do not have a comprehensive cancer plan that could save lives.

　Cancer is a leading cause of death worldwide. The World Health Organization reports 7.6 million people died from cancer in 2008 and almost 13 million new cases of the disease are diagnosed every year.

　WHO says more than two-thirds of these new cases and deaths occur in developing countries and are continuing to increase at an alarming rate. The medical officer in WHO's Department for Chronic Diseases and Health Promotion, Andreas Ullrich, says the future outlook is grim. "With population aging, in particular exposure to major risk factors like tobacco, we expect that over the next 20 years the number of new cases per year will double …We know that physical inactivity, obesity, tobacco use, alcohol use are major risk factors for cancer," said Ullrich. "So, we expect, particularly in the metropolitan areas of the developing world, a major increase in cancer."

　Ullrich says cancer need not be a death sentence. He notes people can prevent up to one-third of deaths by changing their lifestyles. He says modifying risks from tobacco and the harmful use of alcohol, eating better and exercising more to stave off obesity can save lives.

　He notes that some cancers are preventable through vaccinations. "Infections can be prevented through vaccination like hepatitis B, a cause of liver cancer, and we can vaccinate against human papilloma virus," said Ullrich. "We know it is a cause for cervical cancer in women and we have vaccines. And, we hope to prevent cancer. On the other side, the care part is also very promising. We have a huge progress in clinical medicine to treat cancer if detected early." Ullrich says there are many low-cost and effective strategies that countries with limited resources can use to detect and screen various cancers, including cervical and breast cancers.

A WHO survey finds more than half of all countries worldwide lack a comprehensive cancer plan. It says these governments are struggling to prevent cancer and provide treatment and chronic care to patients. Responses from 185 countries reveal major gaps in cancer control planning and services. The survey reveals only 17 percent of the African countries and 27 percent of the low-income countries have control plans to prevent, detect, treat and care for cancer patients. None have a budget to support implementation.

(417 words)

(Voice of America, Feb. 4, 2013)

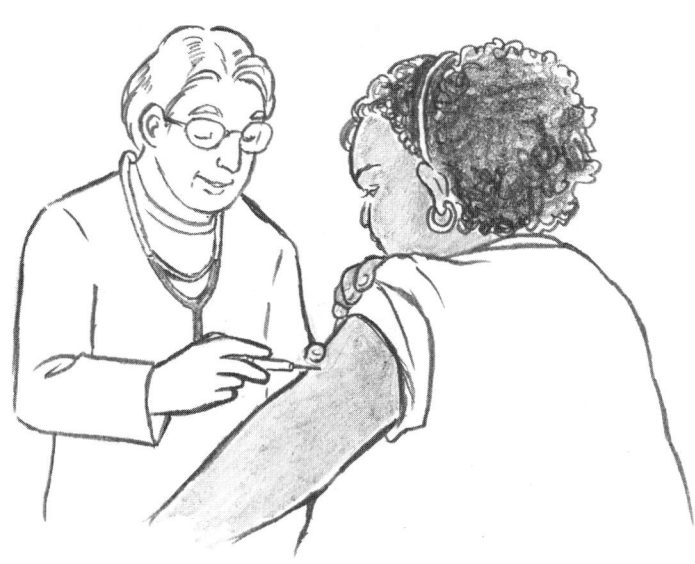

速読をした人は wpm を確認しましょう。

計算式：（あなたのwpm）＝総単語数(417) /（かかった時間(分)）　　あなたのwpm：＿＿＿＿＿wpm

（参考）	1.5 分	278wpm	2 分	209wpm	2.5 分	167wpm
	3 分	139wpm	3.5 分	119wpm	4 分	104wpm
	4.5 分	93wpm	5 分	83wpm	5.5 分	76wpm

内容把握問題　次の１～５の英文が、本文の内容と一致する場合はT、一致しない場合はFを（　）内に記入しましょう。

1. （　）According to the WHO, more than two-thirds of new cancer cases occur in developed countries.
2. （　）Ullrich expects the number of new cancer cases to increase as the population ages.
3. （　）It is thought that all cancer deaths are preventable by making changes in lifestyle.
4. （　）Cervical cancer can be prevented through vaccination against human papilloma virus.
5. （　）Many African countries don't have enough money to carry out cancer control plans.

上記の問題はいくつできましたか？　正解率をあなたのwpmの値にかけてみましょう。

計算式：（あなたの読解効率）＝（あなたのwpm）×（（正答数）/ 5）　　あなたの読解効率：＿＿＿＿＿

語句問題　本文中に出てくる次の１～５の語句とほぼ同じ意味を表すものをa～dの中から１つ選びましょう。

1. comprehensive
   a. understandable　b. inclusive　c. limited　d. selective
2. alarming
   a. startling　b. noisy　c. gradual　d. stable
3. sentence
   a. a set of words　b. punishment　c. a series of signs　d. passage
4. modify
   a. reduce　b. limit　c. qualify　d. alter
5. promising
   a. gifted　b. unfavorable　c. honest　d. hopeful

文法解説【関係代名詞】

関係代名詞は、文と文をつなぐ接続詞と代名詞の働きを兼ね備えています。関係代名詞が導く節に修飾される（代）名詞を先行詞といいます。関係代名詞は、先行詞により異なります。

先行詞	主格	所有格	目的格	
人	who	whose	whom〔who〕	省略可
人以外	which	whose / of which	which	省略可
人・人以外	that	×	that	省略可
なし（先行詞を含む）	what	×	what	

① 先行詞が「人」の場合（who, whose, whom）
　【例】*Those* who drank three to six cups of tea a day had an 11 to 20 percent lower risk of experiencing a stroke.（主格）
　【例】This article was written by *a person* whom〔who〕I worked with.
　※ whom は文語体であり、目的語の働きをする場合でも多くの場合 who が用いられます。

② 先行詞が「人以外」の場合（which, whose）
　【例】The doctor prescribed *medicine* which worked well.

③ 先行詞が「人」または「人以外」の場合（that）
　that は、which の代わりによく使われます。who, whom の代わりに使うこともできますが、人が先行詞の場合には、who, whom のほうが好まれます。
　【例（本文）】More than half of all countries do not have a comprehensive *cancer plan* that could save lives.

④ 先行詞を含んでいる関係代名詞 （what）
　what（= the thing(s) which）は先行詞なしで用い、「こと・もの」と訳します。
　【例】What is important is to prevent cancer.

【関係代名詞の用法：限定用法と継続用法】
関係代名詞には、先行詞を限定する限定用法（先行詞＋関係代名詞）と、先行詞についての説明を追加する継続用法（先行詞＋, 関係代名詞）があります。that は継続用法では用いられません。
　※継続用法の意味：継続用法では、文の途中に挿入されたものでない限り、おもに次の3つの意味があり、接続詞＋代名詞で置き換えることができます。
　　①「・・・して〜」and ＋代名詞　　②「・・・というのも〜」because, for ＋代名詞
　　③「・・・だが〜」but ＋代名詞
　※継続用法の which には、その前の句・節や文の一部または全体を先行詞とする場合があります。
　【例】*Kaori got married*, which surprised us.　＝　Kaori got married and this surprised us.

文法問題 次の1～10の英文の（　）内に入れるのに最も適切なものをa～dの中から1つ選びましょう。

1. He is a doctor (　　　) specializes in treating cancer.
   a. who　　　b. whose　　　c. whom　　　d. which
   ※ specialize in ～：～を専門とする

2. Doctors recommend genetic tests for women (　　　) close relatives have had breast or ovarian cancer.
   a. who　　　b. whose　　　c. whom　　　d. which
   ※ genetic test：遺伝子検査　　ovarian cancer：卵巣がん

3. Pigs have organs (　　　) are similar in both size and shape to those of human's.
   a. who　　　b. whose　　　c. what　　　d. that
   ※ organ：臓器

4. Dr. Yamanaka, (　　　) won the Nobel Prize in Physiology or Medicine, succeeded in generating stem cells from skin tissue.
   a. who　　　b. that　　　c. what　　　d. which
   ※ Nobel Prize in Physiology or Medicine：ノーベル生理学・医学賞　　stem cell：幹細胞
   　skin tissue：皮膚組織

5. Age-related macular degeneration (AMD) is an eye disease (　　　) leads to reduced vision or blindness.
   a. who　　　b. whose　　　c. what　　　d. that
   ※ age-related macular degeneration (AMD)：加齢黄斑変性

6. The number of adults (　　　) have no immunity to rubella is increasing in Japan.
   a. who　　　b. whose　　　c. whom　　　d. which
   ※ immunity：免疫　　rubella：風疹

7. Preventive surgery, (　　　) was a new idea, can lower the odds of getting breast cancer.
   a. who　　　b. that　　　c. what　　　d. which
   ※ preventive surgery：予防手術

8. Doctors tried to determine (　　　) triggers a patient's anaphylactic shock.
   a. who　　　b. that　　　c. what　　　d. which
   ※ anaphylactic shock：アナフィラキシー・ショック

9. Tobacco contains a substance (　　　) causes cancer.
   a. who　　　b. that　　　c. of which　　　d. what

10. The patient (　　　) had made a complete recovery suffered a relapse one month later.
    a. who　　　b. whose　　　c. whom　　　d. what
    ※ recovery：回復　　relapse：再発

英作文 次の1〜5の日本文を英語になおしましょう。

1. 医者は患者の話に耳を傾けなければならない。（what を用いて）
2. 彼女を治療した医者はすぐに回復する（recover）だろうといった。
3. 肺は呼吸をするために使用する器官（organ）だ。
4. 看護師は父親が昏睡状態（in a coma）の息子を励ました（encourage）。
5. 昨日捻挫した（sprain）足首（ankle）を見せてください。

Let's think!

発がん性物質にはどのようなものがあるか調べて、社会・個人としてどのような対処法があるか考えてみましょう。

【例】human papilloma virus, hepatitis B, tobacco, alcohol, asbestos, ultraviolet ray

Let's make a speech!

がんを予防するための生活習慣について、参考文献やインターネットなどを調べてまとめ、英語で3分間のスピーチをしてみましょう。

Column [コラム]　がん

がんは日本人の死亡原因の第1位です。国立がん研究センターの2011年度のデータによると、生涯がん死亡リスクは男性26％、女性16％であり、男性の4人に1人、女性の6人に1人はがんで亡くなっていることになります。

がんの予防、およびがんによる死亡リスクを下げるための方法

①生活習慣の改善

1996年に発表されたアメリカ人のがん死亡原因は、1位 喫煙（30％）、2位 食事（30％）、3位 運動不足（5％）、4位 飲酒（3％）でした。そのため、がんを予防するためには、以下の4点の生活習慣を心がけることが大切です。

1. 喫煙をしない、受動喫煙を避ける
2. 塩分を控え、バランスのよい食事をとる
3. 毎日1時間程度の運動を行い、適正な体重を維持する
4. 過度の飲酒を避ける

②がん検診の受診

医学の進歩により、早期発見であればがんの完治率は上昇しています。2012年6月に、厚生労働省は「5年以内にがん検診の受診率を50％以上とする」という「がん対策推進基本計画」を掲げました。しかし、2009年のOECDの調査によると、例えば子宮頸がん検診の受診率はアメリカ82.6％、イギリス69.8％に比べ、日本は23.7％と低いです。そこで厚生労働省は、20～40歳を対象に、乳がんと子宮頸がんの節目検診（20歳、25歳、30歳、35歳、40歳）には「無料クーポン券」付きのがん検診手帳を配布するなど、がん検診受診率を上げるためのさまざまな取り組みを行っています。

③予防的手術

2013年に、アメリカの人気女優アンジェリーナ・ジョリーが両乳房切除手術・卵巣摘出手術を受け、世界的なニュースになりました。彼女の母親は乳がん・卵巣がんで56歳の若さで亡くなり、彼女自身にも乳がん・卵巣がんを引き起こす可能性のある変形BRCA遺伝子が発見されたのです。彼女の場合、将来乳がんになる可能性は87％、卵巣がんになる可能性は50％以上だったため、予防的手術に踏み切ったといいます。しかし、このような予防的手術は、保険適用外のため、高額な費用がかかるうえ、がんの発症率が0％になるわけではないなどの問題もあります。

Chapter 4　日本人気質もうつ病の原因？

厚生労働省の調査によると、精神疾患により医療機関にかかっている患者数は近年大幅に増加しており、平成23年は320万人と、依然300万人を超えています。なかでも「うつ病」の占める割合は大きく、年間3万人という日本人の自殺の原因ともなっています。しかし、なぜ日本人にうつ病が増えているのでしょうか。そこには、文化的、社会的背景も関係しているようです。

CD Track 05

Depression Is a National Ailment That Demands Open Recognition in Japan

Vocabulary Check（英文を読む前に意味を確認しましょう。）

- depression：うつ病
- ailment：(軽い、または慢性的な) 病気
- public health：公衆衛生
- vascular disease：血管疾患
- prevalence：罹患率
- Alzheimer's disease　アルツハイマー病
- guise：姿、様子
- alcoholism：アルコール依存症
- homelessness：ホームレスの状態
- self-harm：自傷行為
- domestic violence：家庭内暴力
- child abuse：児童虐待
- mood disorder：気分障害
- crux：最も重要な点
- stride：進歩
- general practitioner：一般医
- attribute A to B：AをBのせいにする
- meme：遺伝子のように受け継がれていく社会習慣や文化
- exacerbate：悪化させる
- reticent：多くを語らない
- divulge：明かす
- the Japan Committee for Prevention and Treatment of Depression
  一般社団法人うつ病の予防・治療日本委員会（略称　JCPTD）
- proactive：(行動などが) 先を見越した
- bolster：支える
- self-esteem：自尊心
- astounding：びっくり仰天するような
- let alone ～：～はいうまでもなく
- come to terms with ～：～を甘受する、慣れる
- high-profile：注目を引きがちな
- royalty：皇族
- *Wedge*：株式会社ウェッジが刊行する総合月刊誌
- freelance：自由契約の
- conservatively：控えめにいって
- toll：犠牲
- consecutive：連続した
- dignified self-restraint：威厳のある自制
- prim respectability：きちんとした体面
- compel：強制的に～させる
- de-emphasize：あまり強調しない
- embarrassment：困惑、当惑
- immense：計り知れない
- inflict：苦しめる
- psychiatric disorder：精神障害

・自信のある人は英文をできるだけ速く読み、時間を計ってください。苦手な人はゆっくり読みましょう。

　The greatest public health issue facing the people of Japan today is not cancer. It is not vascular diseases that can cause heart attacks and strokes. It is not the prevalence of Alzheimer's disease in the ever-rising number of the elderly. It is depression in its many forms and guises. Name any significant social problem — alcoholism and other drug-related illnesses, homelessness, teenage pregnancies, self-harm, domestic violence, child abuse, suicide — and you are more than likely to find some form of depression or serious mood disorder as a cause.

　Recognition is the crux of the problem. While big strides have been made in the treatment of depression in Japan over recent years, thanks in part to effective new drugs, the recognition of depression at the primary-care level is inadequate. General practitioners are not sufficiently trained to recognize depression. They too often attribute symptoms to other illnesses. The KITY (keep it to yourself) meme exacerbates this. Japanese tend to be too reticent to divulge their true anxieties to anyone.

Active for the last 40 years, the Japan Committee for Prevention and Treatment of Depression has held countless conferences, meetings and forums for health professionals and the public. The organization is proactive in trying to train doctors to recognize depression when they see it. National broadcaster NHK's educational channel has also had some amazingly frank shows about depression — including one in which female sufferers admitted to having sex with a great number of men in order to bolster their self-esteem. The courage of these women, who appeared under their own names, would be astounding in any country — let alone in Japan, where appearances count for so much.

But Japanese society will not come to terms with depression until very high-profile sufferers — whether royalty, movie stars or politicians — come out from behind the folding screen and openly talk about their illness. Writing in the February issue of the Japanese monthly news and current affairs magazine *Wedge*, freelance journalist Ryutaro Kaibe points out that every year between 800,000 and 1.2 million Japanese quit or stay away from work because of depression. To such costs must be added the human costs of suicides stemming from depression. Conservatively, 30 percent of the annual toll — more than 30,000 dead for 13 consecutive years — is due to depression. Most estimates indicate half, while some go as high as 80 percent to 90 percent.

It may be the sense of dignified self-restraint and prim respectability that compel Japanese people — particularly, as tradition has dictated, women — to de-emphasize their needs and display only the mildest forms of "proper" embarrassment. But when it comes to depression and the immense toll it is inflicting on individuals and society, it is time to abandon these shared virtues and go public. As much as two-thirds of psychiatric disorders go untreated; and only one-fourth of sufferers receive some sort of medical help. This would imply that millions of people are still forced to suffer in silence.

(490 words)

(Japan Times, Feb. 12, 2012)

(Roger Pulvers)

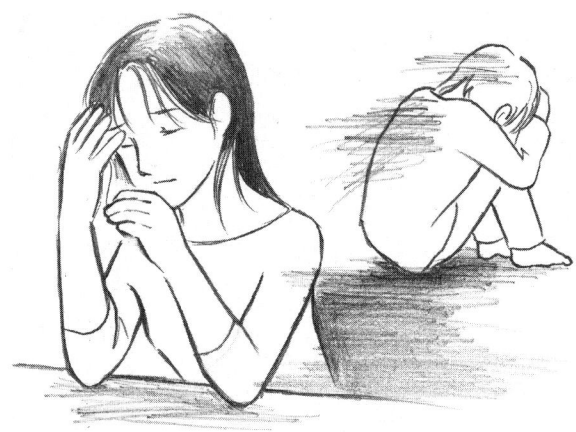

速読をした人は wpm を確認しましょう。

計算式：（あなたの wpm）＝総単語数（490）/（かかった時間（分））　　あなたの wpm：　　　　　wpm

(参考)　2分　245wpm　　　　2.5分　196wpm　　　　3分　163wpm
　　　3.5分　140wpm　　　　4分　123wpm　　　　4.5分　109 wpm
　　　5分　98wpm　　　　5.5分　89wpm　　　　6分　82wpm

内容把握問題　次の１〜５の英文が、本文の内容と一致する場合はT、一致しない場合はFを（ ）内に記入しましょう。

1. （　） The greatest public health issue in Japan is not depression but Alzheimer's disease.
2. （　） Some social problems such as alcoholism and child abuse have nothing to do with depression or mood disorders.
3. （　） Though general practitioners are trained to recognize depression, they sometimes attribute the symptoms to other illness.
4. （　） It is necessary for Japanese people to abandon shared virtues, like KITY, for the proper treatment of depression.
5. （　） It seems that millions of people who have mental disorders receive no medical help.

上記の問題はいくつできましたか？　正解率をあなたの wpm の値にかけてみましょう。

計算式：（あなたの読解効率）＝（あなたの wpm）×（（正答数）/ 5）　　あなたの読解効率：

語句問題　本文中に出てくる次の１〜５の語句とほぼ同じ意味を表すものをa〜dの中から１つ選びましょう。

1. inadequate
　　a. sufficient　　b. competent　　c. not good enough　　d. invaluable
2. keep it to yourself
　　a. keep it a habit　　b. keep it a secret　　c. keep it down　　d. keep it up
3. countless
　　a. a great number of　　b. few　　c. limited　　d. a handful of
4. count
　　a. add up　　b. consider　　c. matter　　d. calculate
5. virtue
　　a. vice　　b. morality　　c. failing　　d. disadvantage

文法解説【関係副詞】

関係副詞は、接続詞＋副詞の働きをして文と文をつなぎます。関係副詞が導く節に修飾される副詞もしくは前置詞＋名詞を先行詞といいます。関係副詞には次の4種類があります。

① **where**（先行詞が「場所」を表す語の場合）
　【例】This is (the place) where Mr. Hattori was shot and killed.
② **when**（先行詞が「時」を表す語の場合）
　【例】He didn't know (the time) when his father would have the operation.
③ **why**（先行詞が reason(s) の場合）
　【例】I couldn't understand (the reason) why the nurse behaved in such a manner.
④ **how**（先行詞は the way ですが、省略します。the way を使う場合は how を省略します。）
　【例】This is how this doctor examines his patients.

　※ the time, the place, the reason などの先行詞は多くの場合省略されます。
　※関係副詞 when, why は省略されることが多いです。（ただし、先行詞も関係副詞も両方とも省略することはできません。）
　※関係副詞は「（適切な）前置詞＋which」に書き換えることができます。
　　例）This is the hospital where I was born. ＝ This is the hospital in which I was born.

【関係副詞の継続用法】
【例（本文）】
　... let alone *in Japan*, where appearances count for so much.
　(= ... let alone *in Japan*, and appearances count for so much there.
　　　　　　　　　　　　　　　　　　　　　　　　　(= *in Japan*)

本文中の関係副詞の前にはコンマがついています。これは継続用法といい、when と where に使われる用法です（why と how に継続用法はありません）。継続用法の場合、いったん文の切れ目があるので、where は、... and there ～（…する。そこでは～）、when は、... and then ～（…する。そのとき～）の意味になります。

文法問題　次の1〜10の英文の（　）内に、適切な関係副詞（when, where, why, how）を入れましょう。

1. I like children. That's (　　　) I became a pediatrician.
   ※ pediatrician：小児科医
2. She was born on the day (　　　) her father died.
3. Tell me the reason (　　　) you became a nurse.
4. Locate sites (　　　) the tumor is bleeding.
   ※ tumor：腫瘍
5. Watch carefully. This is (　　　) the catheter is inserted.
   ※ catheter：カテーテル
6. This is (　　　) my mother was hospitalized five years ago.
7. The doctors didn't know the reason (　　　) the patient suddenly got worse.
8. This is the hospital (　　　) I worked as a resident for three years.
   ※ resident：研修医
9. The day will come (　　　) cancers can be cured.
10. Dr. Marshall experimented on himself by drinking a test tube of bacteria cultured in the stomachs of patients with ulcers. This is (　　　) he showed that bacteria cause gastritis.
    ※ test tube：試験管　　culture：培養する　　ulcer：潰瘍　　gastritis：胃炎

英作文　次の1〜5の日本文を英語になおしましょう。
1. こういうふうにして私は医学を学んだ。
2. 私たちは東京に引っ越して、そこで開業した（open a clinic）。
3. なぜ看護師になったのかと考えるときがある。
4. 人々が心臓病にかかる理由はたくさんある。
5. これが私の父が働いている医療センター（medical center）だ。

Let's think!

あなたはどんなときに「落ち込み」ますか。また、そのような時、どのような方法で気分を変えますか。英語であなたの経験を語ってみましょう。

Let's make a speech!

初期段階でうつ病を正しく診断する方法について、参考文献やインターネットなどを調べてまとめ、英語で3分間のスピーチをしてみましょう。

> **Column [コラム]**
>
> ## 緊急救命室での精神疾患
>
> 病院の緊急救命室（emergency room）にやってくるのは、身体に病気があったり、怪我をしたりした人たちばかりではありません。精神疾患を抱えてやってくる人たちもいます。本章で取り上げたうつ病（depression）のほかにも、パニック発作（panic attack）、境界性パーソナリティ障害（borderline personality disorder）、解離性同一性障害（dissociative identity disorder）、アルコールやドラッグの濫用、双極性障害（bipolar disorder）、統合失調症（schizophrenia）、アルツハイマー型認知症（Alzheimer's dementia）などに苦しむ患者たちがやって来ます。そのあたりは、米国の精神科医 René J. Muller が著した *Psych ER: Psychiatric Patients Come to the Emergency Room*（日本語版は『アメリカ精神科ER　緊急救命室の患者たち』（新興医学出版社））に詳しく描かれています。緊急救命室を訪れた 2000 人以上の患者を診断した同氏の経験にもとづいた 30 数名の患者たちのストーリーです。本章で取り上げた日本の現状と比較して読むと興味深いでしょう。

Chapter 5 エイズ対策は国際的規模で

エイズに苦しむ人々は世界にどれくらいいるのでしょうか？ また対策は十分にとられているのでしょうか？

CD Track 06

Eight Million People Now Being Treated for HIV

Vocabulary Check（英文を読む前に意味を確認しましょう。）

- antiretroviral：抗レトロウイルスの（抗レトロウイルス薬） ▶ immunodeficiency：免疫不全
- The Joint United Nations Program on HIV/AIDS (UNAIDS)：国連共同エイズプログラム
- release：公表する ▶ availability：有効性 ▶ life-saving：救命の ▶ tuberculosis：結核
- malaria：マラリア ▶ likelihood：可能性 ▶ intravenous：静脈内の
- CD4 count：HIVが付着しやすいT4細胞の表面にあるタンパク質の総数
- immune system cell：免疫細胞

・自信のある人は英文をできるだけ速く読み、時間を計ってください。苦手な人はゆっくり読みましょう。

More than eight million people around the world are now receiving antiretroviral drug therapy. That is a twenty percent increase over the past year. All those receiving the treatment have the human immunodeficiency virus, known as HIV.

The Joint United Nations Program on HIV/AIDS (UNAIDS) released a report before the AIDS conference. The report is called "Together We Will End AIDS." It says almost one point four million people were added to the number of people receiving treatment in the last year alone. More than thirty-four million people are now living with HIV. The report says that is the largest number ever, because of the greater availability of life-saving drugs. But about two-point-five million people were newly-infected with the virus last year.

UNAIDS says billions of dollars more will be needed for the fight against HIV/AIDS. The UN group says one point seven million people died from AIDS-related causes last year. That is twenty-four percent fewer deaths than in two thousand five, when the number of deaths was at its highest. Tuberculosis — or TB — is the number one cause of death among people living with HIV. People suffering from HIV/AIDS have weakened natural defenses for fighting disease. That increases their likelihood of getting TB.

People between the ages of fifteen and twenty-four are responsible for forty percent of all new adult HIV infections. Most of those infections are among young women. Studies have shown that many young people do not know how to prevent HIV infection. Many of those infected in parts of Asia and Eastern Europe do not have access to treatment. And infections are increasing among sex workers, men who have sex with men and users of intravenous drugs.

The World Health Organization says developing countries need a full plan of action for treating HIV. WHO officials say some groups of people are still unable to get the treatments they need. Studies have shown that antiretroviral drugs extend the lives of people infected with HIV. The drugs can also prevent infection. This means countries may be able to slow the spread of AIDS. Another part of the fight against HIV/AIDS is the question of when to start treatment. In the early days of antiretrovirals, the drugs were usually given to people when the body's defenses against disease had collapsed. A person's health is measured by the CD4 count. That is the number of immune system cells a person has. The WHO official says many infections could be avoided by giving treatment earlier. Two recent studies have confirmed the effectiveness of what is being called the "treatment as prevention" plan.

　Dr. Hirnschall, director of the World Health Organization's HIV/AIDS Department says it would cost more in the short-term to put more people on antiretrovirals sooner — probably billions more. But he says, in the long-term, the cost will drop and lives will be saved. He also (Dr. Hirnschall) says the World Health Organization is writing rules to help developing countries care for and treat those most at risk of infection.

(503 words)

(Voice of America, Aug. 22, 2012)

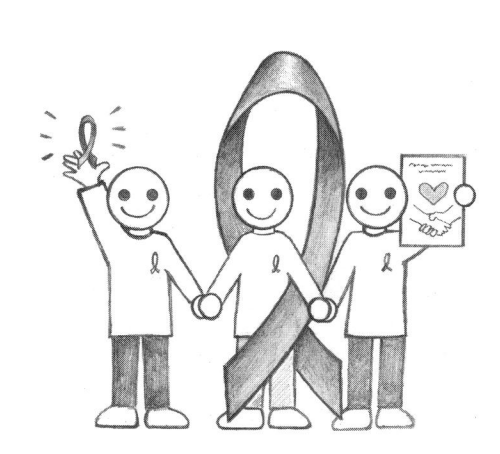

速読をした人は wpm を確認しましょう。

計算式：（あなたのwpm）＝総単語数(503)／（かかった時間(分)）　　　　**あなたのwpm：**　　　　wpm

（参考）	2分	252wpm	2.5分	201wpm	3分	168wpm
	3.5分	144wpm	4分	126wpm	4.5分	112 wpm
	5分	101wpm	5.5分	91wpm	6分	83wpm

内容把握問題　次の1〜5の英文が、本文の内容と一致する場合はT、一致しない場合はFを（　）内に記入しましょう。

1. (　　) There were about one million people who were taking HIV drugs the previous year.
2. (　　) Nearly 34 million people were newly infected with HIV last year.
3. (　　) The number-one cause of death among people with HIV is tuberculosis.
4. (　　) People over 30 are responsible for 40 percent of all new adult HIV infections.
5. (　　) Studies have shown that antiretroviral drugs not only extend the lives of people infected with HIV but also prevent infection.

上記の問題はいくつできましたか？　正解率をあなたのwpmの値にかけてみましょう。

計算式：（あなたの読解効率）＝（あなたのwpm）×（（正答数）/ 5）　　　　**あなたの読解効率：**

語句問題　本文中に出てくる次の1〜5の語句とほぼ同じ意味を表すものをa〜dの中から1つ選びましょう。

1. therapy
    a. treatment　　b. analysis　　c. injection　　d. abuse
2. study
    a. investment　　b. remain　　c. seeking　　d. research
3. defense
    a. weapon　　b. explanation　　c. defect　　d. immunity
4. prevent
    a. advent　　b. avert　　c. defend　　d. pretend
5. effectiveness
    a. inefficiency　　b. success　　c. uselessness　　d. influence

文法解説 【分詞構文】

分詞（現在分詞・過去分詞）が、動詞と接続詞の働きを兼ねて、副詞的に文の情報を補足するものを分詞構文といいます。

① 時：「〜するとき、〜している間に」　省略されている接続詞　when, while, after, before など
　【例】Skiing in Hokkaido, I twisted my ankle.
　　　（= While I was skiing in Hokkaido, I twisted my ankle.）

② 原因・理由：「〜なので」　省略されている接続詞　because, since など
　【例】Understanding what he said, I remained silent.

③ 条件：「〜すれば」　省略されている接続詞　if
　【例】Adding the figure to the list, the total amount will be over 10 million.

④ 譲歩「〜だが、〜だけれども」　省略されている接続詞　although, though など
　【例】Sitting in the sun（= Though I am sitting in the sun), I still feel cold.

⑤　付帯状況
　(1)　2つの動作が同時に行われる場合：「〜しながら」
　【例】The old woman got down from the car, holding on to the driver.
　(2)　動作の連続：「〜して、そして」　省略されている接続詞　and
　【例】Rats caused an outbreak of pneumonic plague, resulting in the deaths of 63 people.

【独立分詞構文】
分詞の意味上の主語が文の主語と一致していない分詞構文を独立分詞構文といいます。この時、分詞の意味上の主語は分詞の直前に主格で置きます。
　【例】My mother being ill, I decided to be a nurse.

【分詞句の否定】
　分詞構文の分詞句の内容を否定する場合には、分詞の直前に not を置きます。
　【例】Not knowing what to say, I left the patient without saying a word.

文法問題　次の 1 ～ 10 の英文を分詞構文を用いて書きかえましょう。

1. While I was walking down the street, I met Dr. Kitano.
2. If all things are equal, the simplest explanation is the best.
3. As the patient is a vegetarian, he doesn't eat any kind of meat.
4. I fell down and struck my head against the door.
5. She entered the consulting room and was accompanied by her mother.
6. Since she was badly injured, she couldn't walk.
7. When he was asked some questions by his proffessor, the student was not able to answer.
8. Though she had a fever, she took the entrance axamination.
9. As it was a fine day, we decided to take the patient for a walk.
10. After they had received their medical check, the astronauts boarded their spacecraft.

　　※ medical check：健康診断　　astronaut：宇宙飛行士

英作文　次の 1 ～ 5 の日本文を分詞構文を用いた英語になおしましょう。

1. 疲れていたので、昨夜は早く寝た。
2. 風邪をひいたので、私は昨日医者にみてもらった。
3. 熱心に勉強したので、その学生は医師国家試験（national exam for medical practitioners）に合格した。
4. どうしてよいかわからなかったので、彼女は看護師に助言を求めた。
5. 主治医を見ると、彼女は微笑んだ。

Let's think!

次のインターネット上のドキュメンタリー番組を観て、感想を英語で話してみましょう。
FRONTLINE: ENDGAME, AIDS IN Black AMERICA
http://www.pbs.org/wgbh/pages/frontline/aids/

Let's make a speech!

死に至る病、エイズを撲滅するにはどうすればよいか。インターネットなどで調べ、あなたの意見を 3 分間でスピーチをしてみましょう。

世界エイズデーとレッドリボン

Column [コラム]

　世界エイズデー（World AIDS Day：12月1日）は、世界レベルでのエイズのまん延防止と患者・感染者に対する差別・偏見の解消を目的に、WHO（世界保健機関）が1988年に制定したもので、毎年12月1日を中心に、世界各国でエイズに関する啓発活動が行われています。

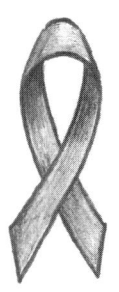

　"レッドリボン（赤いリボン）"は、もともとヨーロッパに古くから伝承される風習のひとつで、病気や事故で人生を全うできなかった人々への追悼の気持ちを表すものでした。

　この"レッドリボン"がエイズのために使われ始めたのは、アメリカでエイズが社会的な問題となってきた1980年代の終わりごろです。このころ、演劇や音楽などで活動するニューヨークのアーティスト達にもエイズがひろがり、エイズに倒れて死亡するアーティスト達が増えていきました。そうした仲間達に対する追悼の気持ちとエイズに苦しむ人々への理解と支援の意思を示すため、"赤いリボン"をシンボルにした運動が始まりました。

　この運動は、その考えに共感した人々によって国境を越えた世界的な運動として発展し、UNAIDS（国連合同エイズ計画）のシンボルマークにも採用されています。レッドリボンは、あなたがエイズに関して偏見をもっていない、エイズとともに生きる人々を差別しないというメッセージなのです。

（参照：厚生労働省ホームページ　http://www.mhlw.go.jp/bunya/kenkou/eizu/）

Chapter 6 「救急ヘリ」と「救急車」どちらを選ぶ？

「ドクターヘリ」や「フライトナース」という言葉を聞いたことがありますか？　欧米諸国では、1970年代から救急医療体制にヘリコプターを導入しています。地理的条件は欧米諸国とは異なりますが、日本でも救命医療の現場に救急ヘリが出動するようになりました。日本の状況を学びましょう。

CD Track 07

Medevac Copters Soon to Cover Entire Nation

Vocabulary Check（英文を読む前に意味を確認しましょう。）

- medevac copter：救急ヘリコプター　　● chopper：ヘリコプター（俗称）
- on standby：待機している　　● subject to ～：～を条件として　　● air ambulance：救急ヘリ
- dispatch：急いで派遣する　　● mechanic：整備士　　● cockpit：コックピット、操縦室
- on board：搭乗して　　● emergency care：救急医療　　● casualty：負傷者　　● transportation：輸送
- be critical to ～：～に欠かせない　　● bleed internally：内出血する　　● due to ～：～が原因で
- cardiac rupture：心破裂　　● trauma care：外傷ケア　　● diagnose：診断する　　● first aid：応急処置
- take into consideration ～：～を考慮する　　● level of consciousness：意識レベル
- cost-effectiveness：費用対効果
- Emergency Medical Network of Helicopter and Hospital：特定非営利活動法人（NPO）救急ヘリ病院ネットワーク（略称 HEM-Net）

・自信のある人は英文をできるだけ速く読み、時間を計ってください。苦手な人はゆっくり読みましょう。

　At Nippon University's Chiba Hokuso Hospital in Inzai, Chiba Prefecture, a white chopper is on standby at the heliport.* Subject to weather, the air ambulance can be dispatched between 8:30 a.m. and 30 minutes before sunset. With a pilot and mechanic in the cockpit, the helicopter usually takes off with a doctor and a nurse on board to provide emergency care during patient airlifts. In cases involving several casualties, the helicopter takes off with two doctors on board.

　Unlike land transportation, where emergency vehicles are often delayed by traffic, helicopters usually arrive at the indicated time. Professor Kunihiro Mashiko, head of the Emergency Medical Care Center of Hokuso Hospital, says that receiving emergency care within 30 to 40 minutes of receiving a severe injury is critical to survival. In fact, Hokuso Hospital had a case in which a person bleeding internally due to a cardiac rupture survived thanks to the prompt treatment and transport, as well as emergency surgery at the hospital. Critical to the entire process was the doctor aboard the helicopter, who accurately identified the cause of the internal bleeding upon arrival at the pickup site. That, Dr. Mashiko insists, illustrates the importance of dispatching not just any doctor, but specialists in emergency medicine and trauma care. Highly specialized knowledge in

36

emergency medical care is needed because the air ambulance physician must decide — after diagnosing the nature and extent of injury and giving first aid — the best medical institution to take the patient for the treatment required.

Providing expert medical care quickly to the severely injured or patients experiencing life-threatening heart attacks or strokes not only greatly increases survival rates, it helps save money as well. A team led by Takuhiro Yamaguchi, a professor of medical statistics at Tohoku University, conducted a comparative study of people injured in traffic accidents and were taken to one of four hospitals that offer air ambulance services. The study covered 120 patients airlifted to hospitals and 111 who were taken in ground vehicles. The team took into consideration factors that might affect the pace of recovery, such as age, level of consciousness, blood pressure and the extent of the injuries. The analysis showed that the number of days hospitalized was four to 18 days fewer for the patients transported on board a helicopter than those transported by ordinary ambulance. Medical expenses were also lower for the airlifted cases, highlighting the cost-effectiveness of helicopters in emergency medical care.

This year will mark the start of an air ambulance service in Akita and Mie prefectures. Many regions are jointly covered by air ambulance programs for more than one prefecture. Takaji Kunimatsu, president of the Emergency Medical Network of Helicopter and Hospital, stresses that it is vital to enhance the quality of air ambulances as part of medical care and address safety issues to ensure continued operation of air ambulances without accident. The network organizes field training for air ambulance personnel as well as workshops to raise awareness of flight safety issues.

(479 words)

(The Japan Times, Feb. 22, 2012)

(共同通信配信)

＊オリジナル出典通りの名称で記載しているが、正しくは Nippon Medical School's ChibaHokusoh Hospital である。

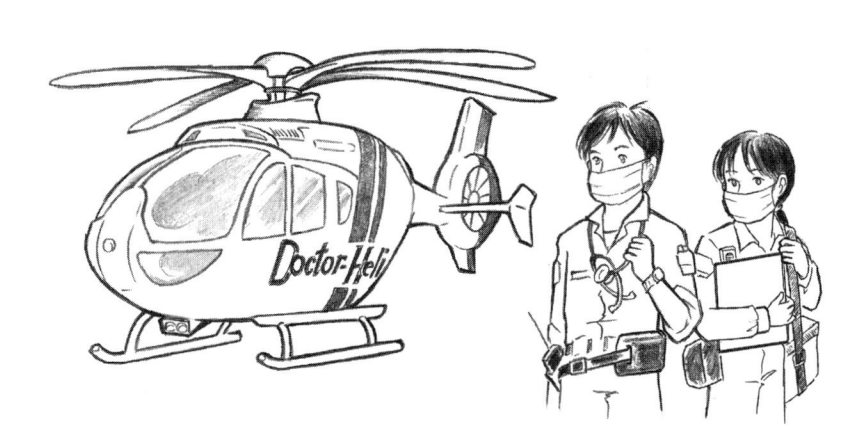

速読をした人は wpm を確認しましょう。

計算式：（あなたの wpm）＝総単語数（479）／（かかった時間（分））　　　あなたの wpm：　　　　　　wpm

（参考）
	2 分	240wpm	2.5 分	192wpm	3 分	160wpm
	3.5 分	137wpm	4 分	120wpm	4.5 分	106wpm
	5 分	96wpm	5.5 分	87wpm	6 分	80wpm

内容把握問題　次の 1 〜 5 の英文が、本文の内容と一致する場合は T、一致しない場合は F を（　）内に記入しましょう。

1. (　　) The advantage of air ambulance service is that it avoids traffic delays.
2. (　　) Air ambulances always carry only one doctor and two nurses to emergencies.
3. (　　) It is necessary for critical patients to receive emergency care within 30 to 40 minutes after being severely injured.
4. (　　) Patients transported by air ambulance are hospitalized longer than those transported by ordinary ambulance.
5. (　　) It is extremely important to think carefully about the safety of air ambulances.

上記の問題はいくつできましたか？　正解率をあなたの wpm の値にかけてみましょう。

計算式：（あなたの読解効率）＝（あなたの wpm）×（（正答数）／ 5）　　　あなたの読解効率：

語句問題　本文中に出てくる次の 1 〜 5 の語句とほぼ同じ意味を表すものを a 〜 d の中から 1 つ選びましょう。

1. provide
   a. show　　　b. send　　　c. get　　　d. give
2. surgery
   a. operation　　　b. treatment　　　c. diagnosis　　　d. examination
3. extent (of injury)
   a. length　　　b. color　　　c. degree　　　d. characteristic
4. highlight
   a. play down　　　b. emphasize　　　c. ignore　　　d. neglect
5. region
   a. area　　　b. population　　　c. institution　　　d. hospital

文法解説【分詞】

動詞の性質（補語や目的語をとる）をもちながら形容詞の働きを有するものを分詞といいます。そのため、分詞は名詞を修飾したり、補語となったりすることができます。分詞には現在分詞（動詞の原形に -ing をつけたもの）と過去分詞（動詞の原形に -ed をつけた規則的なものと、不規則変化をするものとがある）があります。

【現在分詞と過去分詞の使い分け】
「〜している、〜する」という意味を表す時は現在分詞を用います。
「〜される、〜された」という意味を表す時は過去分詞を用います。

【限定用法】
分詞が名詞を修飾する用法を限定用法といいます。現在分詞・過去分詞1語で名詞や代名詞を修飾する場合は、原則として分詞を名詞や代名詞の前に置きますが、ほかの語句と一緒になった場合は、分詞句は名詞・代名詞の後に置かれます。

（1）現在分詞・現在分詞句【例（本文）】
　　In *cases* involving several casualties
　　a person bleeding internally
　　patients experiencing life-threatening heart attacks or strokes

（2）過去分詞・過去分詞句【例（本文）】
　　a team led by Takuhiro Yamaguchi, a professor of medical statistics at Tohoku University
　　people injured in traffic accidents
　　those transported by ordinary ambulance

【叙述用法】
分詞が、動詞や目的語の補語になる用法を叙述用法といいます。この場合、原則として、第2文型もしくは第5文型となります。
　【例】The patient seemed so disappointed after the physical examination.（disappointed が補語⇒第2文型）
　　　　The doctor kept me waiting for about one hour.（waiting が補語⇒第5文型）

文法問題　次の1〜10の英文の（　）内から、最も適切な語を選びましょう。

1. The offspring of all the rats (expose / exposing / exposed) to nicotine showed signs of asthma.
   ※ offspring：子孫　　nicotine：ニコチン　　asthma：喘息
2. The doctor carried out clinical tests (use / using / used) iPS cells.
   ※ clinical test：臨床試験　　iPS cell：iPS 細胞
3. The chemical (contain / containing / contained) in the food might be harmful to health.
4. The bacteria (make / making / made) the patient sick are only weakened, not killed.
5. The number of people (suffer / suffering / suffered) from depression has been increasing.
6. Antibiotic residues (leave / leaving / left) in meat and animal products can lead to drug resistance in humans.
   ※ antibiotic：抗生物質（の）　　residue：残留物質　　drug resistance：薬物耐性
7. The nurse smiled at the baby (sleep / sleeping / slept) in the cradle.
   ※ cradle：ゆりかご
8. The doctor looked so (exhaust / exhausting / exhausted) after the operation.
9. Patients (recover / recovering / recovered) from organ transplants rely on effective antibiotics to fight off infections.
   ※ organ transplant：臓器移植
10. Obstetric fistula can occur during (prolong / prolonging / prolonged) hard labor in childbirth.
    ※ obstetric fistula：産科瘻孔　　labor：陣痛

英作文　次の1〜5の日本文を英語になおしましょう。

1. 一人暮らしをする老人の数が増えてきている。
2. 生命を脅かす病気に苦しんでいる人々は、深刻なストレスにさらされている（be exposed to ～）。
3. 爆発（explosion）のあと救急車で搬送された2人の作業員は、到着時すでに死亡していた。
4. 政府に選ばれた医療チームは、臨床心理士（clinical psychologist）と精神科医（psychiatrist）を含んでいた。
5. 救急ヘリ搬送された人々のほうが生存率（survival rate）が高いということを示すデータがある。

Let's think!

あなたの町ではドクターヘリが導入されていますか？ インターネットなどで調べてみましょう。

Let's make a speech!

世界のドクターヘリについて調べ、英語で3分間のスピーチをしてみましょう。

Column [コラム] 日本のドクターヘリはこれから？

　日本では、2007年にようやく国会で「救急医療用ヘリコプターを用いた救急医療の確保に関する特別措置法」が成立し、ドクターヘリが全国各地に配備されるようになりましたが、欧米諸国では、1970年代から救急医療用ヘリコプターが導入されています。ドイツでは、高速道路（アウトバーン）における死亡者数を減少させるため、医師が搭乗したヘリコプターを高速道路上に着陸させ、救命率の向上に成功しました。スイスでは、山岳救助活動でヘリコプターが用いられてきました。米国では、朝鮮戦争やベトナム戦争時に、前線の負傷兵を医療機関に搬送するためにヘリコプターの活用がはじまりました。本章のタイトルに出てくる medevac という語は、おもに軍事用語として使われますが、medical（医療の）＋ evacuation（撤退）が語源で、最初にこの語が使われたのは1966年です。ただし米国の場合、救急医療用ヘリコプターに搭乗するのは医師ではなく、フライトナース（flight nurse）とよばれる看護師であることがほとんどです。したがって、米国では *Trauma Junkie: Memoirs of an Emergency Flight Nurse*（『救命フライトナース物語』（成美堂））のようなストーリーがありますが、ドクターヘリに関するストーリーはみつかりません。ほかにも、オーストラリアの救急医療用ヘリコプターに搭乗する医師の姿を描いたものに *Helicopter Rescue: The True Story of Australia's First Full-Time Chopper Doctor*（日本語版は『ドクターヘリ 救命飛行』（医歯薬出版））があります。

Chapter 7　ハンズオンリーCPRであなたも人命が救えます

CPR（cardiopulmonary resuscitation）「心肺蘇生術」とは、心臓停止後の心肺機能を蘇らせる措置のことです。CPRといえば、「口移し式の人工呼吸」や「心臓マッサージ」をイメージする人が多いのではないでしょうか。運転免許取得のために自動車学校の講習会などで、人形を相手に訓練したことがある人もいるでしょう。最新のCPRはどうなっているのでしょうか？

CD Track 08

Hands-Only CPR Is a Simpler Way to Save Lives

Vocabulary Check（英文を読む前に意味を確認しましょう。）

- cardiopulmonary resuscitation（CPR）：心肺蘇生　● brain damage：脳損傷
- medical help：医療救助（者）　● the American Heart Association：米国心臓協会（学会）
- simplify：簡素化する　● call for：提唱する　● hands-only：両手だけの
- collapse：倒れる、虚脱する　● unconscious：意識不明の　● cardiac arrest：心停止
- compression：圧迫　● organ：臓器　● rescue breathing：人工呼吸
- drowning：溺水、溺れること

・自信のある人は英文をできるだけ速く読み、時間を計ってください。苦手な人はゆっくり読みましょう。

　　If a person's heart stops, would you know how to perform CPR? CPR, or cardiopulmonary resuscitation, can save a life and reduce the risk of brain damage from loss of oxygen. With traditional CPR, you give two breaths to force air into the lungs. Then you push hard on the chest thirty times. You repeat these two steps until the victim wakes up or medical help arrives.

　　But people may worry about getting sick from blowing into a stranger's mouth. Also, the training is easy to forget, especially during an emergency. And those without training may not do anything for fear that they will do something wrong. So in 2008 the American Heart Association simplified its guidelines.

　　The group now calls for hands-only CPR for adults who suddenly collapse. Here is how it works: A person has collapsed unconscious on the ground. The victim has lost color in the face and does not appear to be breathing. These are signs of cardiac arrest. This is the time to begin CPR. Place your hands, one on top of the other, on the center of the chest. Push hard and fast. Aim for a rate of about one hundred compressions each minute. Chest compressions keep the blood flowing to the brain, heart and other organs.

　　Guidelines from 2005 said only untrained people should use hands-only CPR. Those with training were told to use traditional CPR. But now the heart association says everyone should use hands-only CPR unless they feel strong about their ability to do rescue breathing. The guidelines were updated after three studies showed that the hands-only method was just as effective as traditional CPR. Scientists say enough oxygen remains in a person's system for several minutes after breathing stops.

　But the experts say you should still use traditional CPR with a combination of breaths and compressions on babies and children. Traditional CPR should also be used for adults found already unconscious and not breathing normally. And traditional CPR should be used for any victims of drowning or collapse from breathing problems. These are all examples where CPR with mouth-to-mouth breathing may be more helpful than hands-only CPR. Because there are many of these cases, people should still learn CPR with mouth-to-mouth.

〈384 words〉
（Voice of America, May 19, 2009）

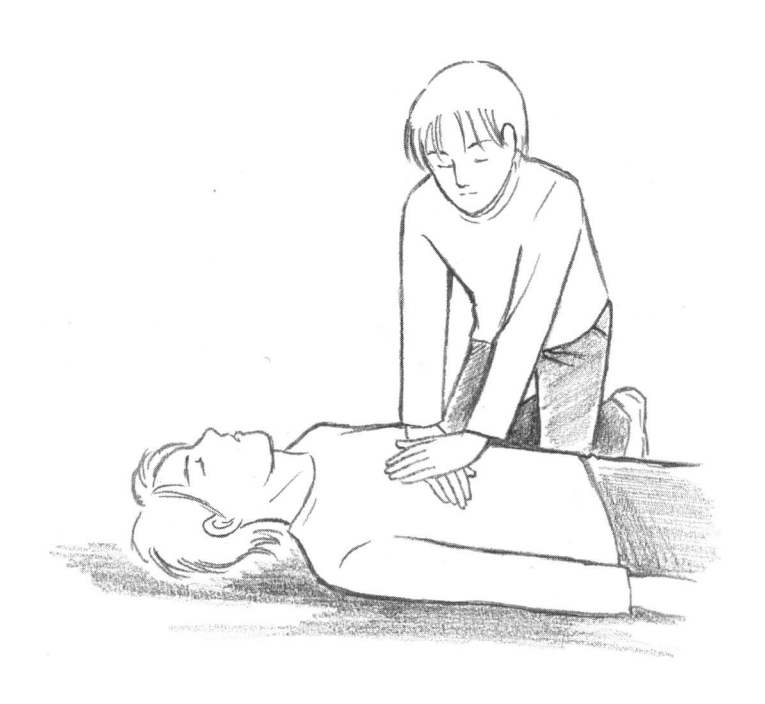

速読をした人は wpm を確認しましょう。

計算式：（あなたの wpm）＝総単語数(384) /（かかった時間(分)）　　　あなたの wpm：　　　　　　　wpm

(参考)　2分　192wpm　　　2.5分　154wpm　　　3分　128wpm
　　　　3.5分　110wpm　　　4分　　96wpm　　　4.5分　85wpm
　　　　5分　　77wpm　　　5.5分　70wpm

内容把握問題　次の1～5の英文が、本文の内容と一致する場合はT、一致しない場合はFを（　）内に記入しましょう。

1. (　　) CPR can reduce the risk of brain damage from loss of blood.
2. (　　) Hands-only CPR is for adults who suddenly fall down.
3. (　　) Three studies have shown that hands-only CPR is less effective than traditional CPR.
4. (　　) Traditional CPR, with mouth-to-mouth breathing and chest compressions, should be used for babies and children.
5. (　　) Traditional CPR should be used for anyone with breathing problems.

上記の問題はいくつできましたか？　正解率をあなたの wpm の値にかけてみましょう。

計算式：（あなたの読解効率）＝（あなたの wpm）×((正答数) / 5)　　　あなたの読解効率：

語句問題　本文中に出てくる次の1～5の語句とほぼ同じ意味を表すものをa～dの中から1つ選びましょう。

1. victim
    a. sufferer　　　b. survivor　　　c. attacker　　　d. loser
2. stranger
    a. audience　　　b. unusual person　　　c. unknown person　　　d. acquaintance
3. association
    a. society　　　b. college　　　c. physician　　　d. system
4. update
    a. innovate　　　b. stick　　　c. outdate　　　d. stand out
5. combination
    a. separation　　　b. mixture　　　c. distinction　　　d. division

文法解説【不定詞】

to +動詞の原形〜の形で、名詞・形容詞・副詞の働きをするものを、不定詞といいます。

① **名詞的用法**　名詞と同様、主語、補語、目的語として用いられます。
It is very important to perform CPR.
※ It is +□+ (for / of +人) + to +動詞の原形〜．の構文では、形式主語の it は、「to +動詞の原形〜」の内容をさします。

② **形容詞的用法**　形容詞と同様、名詞を修飾します。
He has the ability to perform CPR.

③ **副詞的用法**　副詞と同様、動詞、形容詞、副詞を修飾します。
（1）　目的「〜するために」
She performed CPR to save his life.
（2）　感情の原因・理由「〜して…」
I am happy to hear that the mother and her baby will be discharged from the hospital within a few days.
（3）　結果「…その結果〜」
My grandfather lived to be 90.
（4）　判断の根拠「〜するとは」
He is stupid to say such a thing to his patient.
（5）　限定「〜するのは（が）」
※この用法は、easy, difficult, bad, impossible, dangerous, comfortable などの形容詞が to 不定詞の前に来る場合に多くみられます。
This river is dangerous to swim in.

【不定詞句の否定】

不定詞句の内容を否定する場合には、不定詞の直前に not をおきます。
The patient decided not to have an operation.

【原形不定詞】

原形不定詞：使役動詞、知覚動詞の場合は、目的語のあとに to 不定詞ではなく、原形不定詞（=動詞の原形）がきます。（「使役動詞＋ O ＋動詞の原形」、「知覚動詞＋ O ＋動詞の原形」）
Pepper makes us sneeze.（使役動詞）
I saw a lady collapse on the train.（知覚動詞）

文法問題 次の1～10の英文の下線部が、名詞的用法（A）、形容詞的用法（B）、副詞的用法（C）のどれか答えましょう。

1. I am sorry to hear of his illness. （ ）
2. This is the time to begin CPR. （ ）
3. With traditional CPR, you give two breaths to force air into the lungs. （ ）
4. Hands-only CPR is a simpler way to save lives. （ ）
5. The training is easy to forget, especially during an emergency. （ ）
6. To limit the spread of resistant infections, experts recommend wider use of routine immunizations.
（ ）

　　※ resistant infection：（薬剤）耐性感染症　　immunization：免疫付与、予防接種

7. It is hard for patients to manage all medications given to them. （ ）
8. The technique will allow surgeons to distinguish cancer cells from healthy brain cells at the microscopic level. （ ）

　　※　surgeon：外科医　　microscopic：顕微鏡の

9. People in that country may not be able to afford the transportation costs to get to healthcare clinics.
（ ）
10. I found it difficult to work at the hospital. （ ）

英作文 次の1～5の日本文を英語になおしましょう。

1. 医師の予約をいただきたいのですが。（would like to を用いて）
2. 君は医者に診てもらう必要がある。（It … to ～を用いて）
3. 風邪をひかないように気を付けてください。
4. その患者は気難しい人だ。（please（動詞）を用いて）
5. 医者は彼女に絶対安静にする（take a complete rest）ように忠告した。

Let's think!

下のサイトで Hands-only CPR の実際を見て、手順や留意点を確認しましょう。
TWO STEPS TO STAYING ALIVE（American Heart Association）
http://www.heart.org/HEARTORG/CPRAndECC/HandsOnlyCPR/Hands-Only-CPR_UCM_440559_SubHomePage.jsp

Let's make a speech!

目の前で人が倒れ、意識を失い、呼吸をしていないようなら、あなたはどうしますか？
その場の状況を心に描き、どのような応急手当をすべきか英語で3分間のスピーチをしてみましょう。

> **Column**
> [コラム]
>
> ## CPRのA-B-C
>
> 　心肺蘇生術のA-B-Cといえば、以前は、気道確保（Airway）、（人工）呼吸（mouth-to-mouth Breathing）、心臓マッサージ（chest Compressions）でしたが、米国心臓協会（American Heart Association）の2010年ガイドラインでは、一般的に大人に対しては、順番が変わって、C-A-Bを推奨しています。
>
> 各国言語によるハイライト版はこちら↓です。
> http://www.heart.org/HEARTORG/CPRAndECC/Science/Guidelines/Guidelines-Highlights_UCM_317219_SubHomePage.jsp

Chapter 8　災害医療には心のケアも並行して

地震、津波、洪水など大災害にあった人たちの怪我や病気の治療は、緊急を要する医療行為です。しかし、家族や友人を失い、自宅や勤め先の損壊によって生活基盤を奪われ、避難生活を余儀なくされている被災者のメンタルケアも必要です。東日本大震災を契機に、日本でも災害後のメンタルケア・システムの構築が求められています。

CD Track 09

Mental Health Must Match Post-3/11 Recovery

Vocabulary Check（英文を読む前に意味を確認しましょう。）

- trillion：兆　　● robust：力強い　　● urgency：緊急（性）　　● survivor：生存者
- reconstruction：復興　　● furnish：供給する　　● ramification：派生する問題
- well-being：幸福、健康
- Plan Japan：発展途上国の子どもたちの生活環境改善を目的として1937年設立された非営利の国際的民間団体「プラン」の日本支部。「プランジャパン」は「プラン」の一員として、開発途上国の子どもたちの支援を行っているが、災害や紛争被害の復興活動にも取り組んでいる。
- flush：水をどっと流す　　● be scared to ～：～におびえる
- alcohol and gambling addiction：アルコール中毒やギャンブル中毒　　● psycho-social：心理社会的な
- psychiatrist：精神科医　　● clinical psychologist：臨床心理士　　● sentiment：感情、気持ち
- humanitarian　人道主義的な

・自信のある人は英文をできるだけ速く読み、時間を計ってください。苦手な人はゆっくり読みましょう。

　For thousands of tsunami-affected people, life has not moved on since 3/11 as they try to come to terms with their loss. Earthquake, tsunami and the fear of nuclear radiation has put a significant part of the population under stress.

　Japan's decision to spend 13 trillion yen (167 billion dollars) over five years for recovery is a robust response. The urgency to return to business is evident, and core priorities have been set around economic revival and economic benefits. Missing, however, from the discussion is the pressing human needs of survivors. The emotional impact of tsunami on survivors cannot be addressed by rapid reconstruction and physical recovery alone.

　Mental health professionals readily furnish data to show how — years after the 1995 Kobe earthquake, which killed more than 6,000 people — the number of psychological cases continued to rise. They fear that if the emotional needs of affected people are not addressed immediately, there could be long-term ramifications for the general psychological well-being of those at risk, especially children.

　Child rights organization Plan Japan's experience of reaching thousands of tsunami survivors in the past year confirms this assessment. The organization has come across disturbing stories of children playing tsunami games or being scared to flush toilets as it reminds them of tsunami waves. Psychologists working with Plan Japan have reported cases of grown-up children showing anxiety, wetting beds and adults going through depression and some even developing alcohol and gambling addictions.

　Emotional support or psycho-social care is often neglected in disaster response, yet it is among the most basic needs of disaster survivors. It is vital for affected people to be able to relate to and deal with their circumstances. Simple things such as group activities, games or getting people to talk to each other can play a significant role in the healing process. Best still, expressing emotions and sharing feelings can prevent high-risk people from advancing to stages where they require specialized mental health care involving psychiatrists and clinical psychologists.

　The events of 3/11, however, have exposed a worrying neglect of emotional well-being in Japanese society, a sentiment echoed by mental health experts who fear that things could get worse. As the world's third largest economy races for rapid rebuilding and reconstruction, it must not lose sight of survivors' emotional well-being. It is a challenge and a humanitarian need that must be met. For Japan's recovery to be successful, it must be matched in mind.

(404 words)

(The Japan Times, Mar. 9, 2012)

(Davinder Kumar)

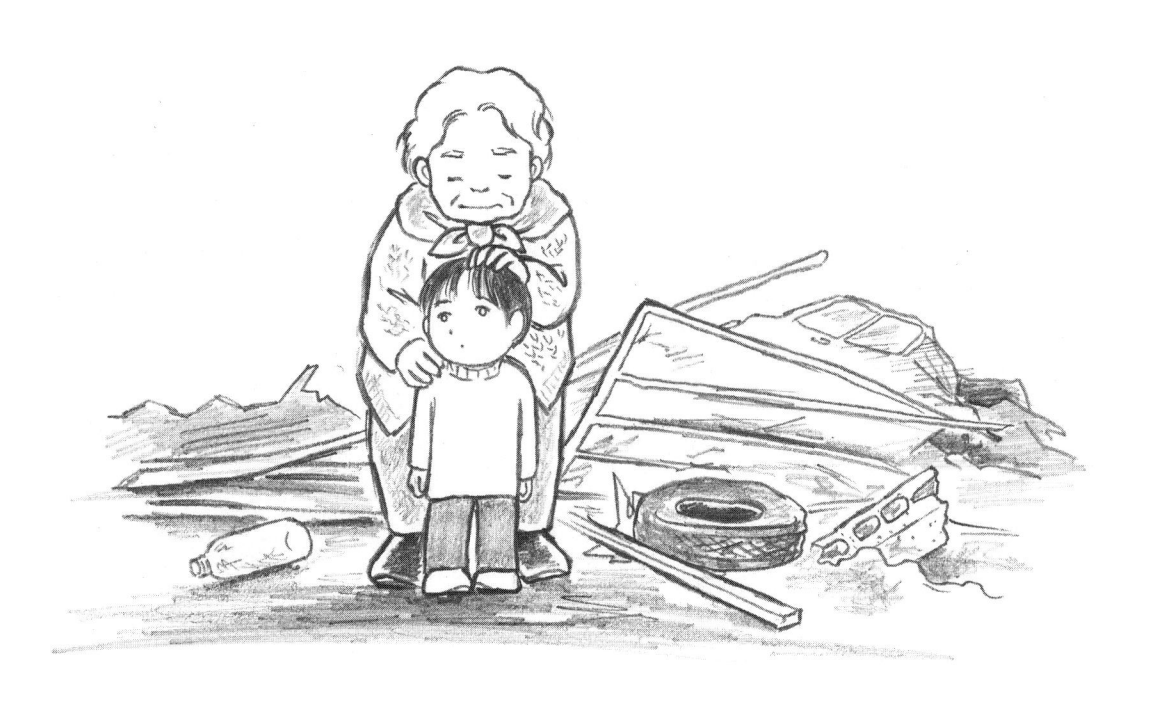

速読をした人は wpm を確認しましょう。

計算式：（あなたのwpm）＝総単語数(403) /（かかった時間(分)）　　　あなたのwpm：　　　　　wpm

(参考)　2分　202wpm　　　　2.5分　161wpm　　　　3分　134wpm
　　　　3.5分　115wpm　　　　4分　101wpm　　　　4.5分　90wpm
　　　　5分　81wpm　　　　　5.5分　73wpm

内容把握問題　次の1〜5の英文が、本文の内容と一致する場合はT、一致しない場合はFを（　）内に記入しましょう。

1. (　　) The Japanese government decided to spend 13 trillion yen, not only for the reconstruction of Tohoku District but also for emotional care for disaster survivors.
2. (　　) More than 6,000 people were killed by the 1995 Kobe earthquake.
3. (　　) Many adults are scared to flush toilets as it reminds them of tsunami waves.
4. (　　) Emotional support is one of the most basic needs of disaster survivors, although it is often neglected just after disasters.
5. (　　) For Tohoku's true recovery, it is crucial to continue psychological support for survivors along with economic reconstruction.

上記の問題はいくつできましたか？　正解率をあなたのwpmの値にかけてみましょう。

計算式：（あなたの読解効率）＝（あなたのwpm）×（（正答数）/ 5）　　　あなたの読解効率：

語句問題　本文中に出てくる次の1〜5の語句とほぼ同じ意味を表すものをa〜dの中から1つ選びましょう。

1. significant
    a. supportive　　b. important　　c. effective　　d. meaningless
2. evident
    a. primary　　b. obvious　　c. doubtful　　d. current
3. priority
    a. promotion　　b. progress　　c. procedure　　d. precedence
4. impact
    a. influence　　b. excitement　　c. factor　　d. situation
5. anxiety
    a. confidence　　b. terror　　c. loneliness　　d. worry

文法解説　【動名詞】

動詞の ing 形で、動詞の性質を持ちながら名詞の働きをするものを動名詞といいます。動名詞（句）は名詞と同様に、主語・目的語・補語・前置詞の目的語になります。

① **主語になる場合**
　【例（本文）】<u>Expressing emotions and sharing feelings</u> can prevent high-risk people from advancing to worse stages.

② **補語になる場合**
　【例】The doctor's dream is <u>presenting his paper</u> at the international conference.

③ **目的語になる場合**
　（1）動詞の目的語
　【例】Do you mind <u>going to the hospital with me</u>?
　※動名詞だけを目的語にとる動詞
　　enjoy, stop, finish, mind, admit, avoid, consider, deny, escape, give up, put off, postpone など。

　（2）前置詞の目的語
　【例（本文）】Plan Japan's experience of <u>reaching thousands of tsunami survivors in the past year</u> confirms this assessment.

④ **動名詞の意味上の主語**
動名詞の意味上の主語は、名詞もしくは代名詞の所有格（または目的格）を動名詞の ing 形の直前に置きます。
　【例（本文）】The organization has come across disturbing stories of <u>children</u> <u>playing</u> tsunami games or <u>being scared</u> to flush toilets as it reminds them of tsunami waves. Psychologists working with Plan Japan have reported cases of grown-up <u>children</u> <u>showing</u> anxiety or <u>wetting</u> beds, and <u>adults</u> <u>going</u> through depression, <u>some</u> even <u>developing</u> alcohol and gambling addictions.

⑤ **動名詞を用いた慣用表現**

there is no ～ing（～できない）	it is no use ～ing（～しても無駄だ）
be worth ～ing（～する価値がある）	how about ～ing（～するのはどうですか）
feel like ～ing（～したい気がする）	cannot help ～ing（～せずにはいられない）
it goes without saying that …（～はいうまでもない）	
on ～ing（～するとすぐに）	in ～ing（～する時に）
look forward to ～ing（～するのを楽しみにしている）	

文法問題

A 次の1〜5の英文の（ ）内の語を適切な形になおしましょう。

1. Scientists have moved a step closer to (develop) a universal vaccine against seasonal influenza.
   ※ universal vaccine：万能ワクチン　　seasonal influenza：季節性インフルエンザ
2. One study found that a number of stroke patients stop (take) their pills within three months after having a stroke.
3. Surgeons need better tools for (visualize) tumors during surgery.
4. (Read) in bed is not good for your eyes.
5. Naps play a critical role in (enhance) learning in young children.

B 日本語を参考に、次の1〜5の英文の（ ）内に適語を入れましょう。

1. その知らせを聞いたとたん、彼は青くなった。
   (　　　　　)(　　　　　　) the news, he turned pale.
2. 私は彼がすぐによくなると確信している。
   I am sure of (　　　　　)(　　　　　　) better soon.
3. 過去のことをくよくよしても無駄だ。
   It is no (　　　　　)(　　　　　　) about the past.
4. 夏の暑いときには、食べる気がしない。
   I don't feel (　　　　　)(　　　　　　) much during the height of summer.
5. 健康が富に勝ることはいうまでもない。
   It goes (　　　　　)(　　　　　　) that health is more important than wealth.

英作文　　次の1〜5の日本文を英語になおしましょう。

1. たばこは2年前にやめた。
2. 第一段階は、医学部（medical college）に入ることだ。（動名詞を用いて）
3. その患者は家族に会うことを楽しみにしている。（look forward to 〜 ing を用いて）
4. 明日何が起こるかわからない。（There is no 〜 ing を用いて）
5. 私は一度その患者に会ったことを覚えている。

Let's think!

次の表の数字を見て、「震災関連死」の問題について考えてみましょう。

The Number of Deaths Related to the Great East Japan Earthquake

Prefecture	Total Number of deaths	1 week after disaster	1 week to 1 month	1 month to 3 months	3 month to 6 months	6 months to 1 year	Over 1 year
Iwate	389	82	115	109	47	28	8
Miyagi	862	228	323	205	74	23	9
Fukushima	1,383	105	239	319	284	307	129
Ibaragi	41	19	12	5	4	1	0
Chiba	4	2	1	0	1	0	0
Others	9	4	3	1	0	0	1
Total	2,688	440	693	639	410	359	147

Complied by the Reconstruction Agency (figures as of March 31, 2013)

Let's make a speech!

次の問について、自分の考えを英語でスピーチしてみましょう。
What do you think is necessary to support people who suffer from hardship and mental stress after surviving the earthquake and tsunami?

Column [コラム] 大災害の後は継続的な心身のケア体制が必要

　復興庁は、東日本大震災以後、避難所生活でのストレスや疲労などで死亡した「震災関連死」が2013年3月31日現在、2600人を超えたことを発表しました。「関連死」の概念は、1995年の阪神大震災で初めて導入され、このときの死者6434人のうち921人（14％）が関連死と認められました。また、2004年の新潟県中越地震では、死者68人中52人（76％）が関連死でした。多くは、避難所生活や移動中の疲労が原因とされますが、ストレスによる体調不良が原因の死亡や自殺も少なくなかったといわれています。

　阪神大震災では、被災者の1割が1年後も睡眠障害などの不調を訴え、さらにその後PTSD（心的外傷後のストレス障害）に苦しむ人も出てきました。とくに、子供たちに関しては、心の問題がピークを迎えたのは3年後であったと報告されています。東日本大震災においても、震災1年を過ぎたころから、子供たちの「心の傷」が、不眠、不登校、過緊張、イライラ、落ち着きのなさなどの現象として、表面化してきました。

　大災害のときには、まず目の前の傷病者の治療に全力を尽くさなければなりませんが、生き残った被災者の体調や精神状態にも目を向けていく必要があります。大災害後のトラウマ反応に対処するために、治療体制の確立や、専門家の養成、拠点施設・病院の確立なども進めていかなければなりません。

Chapter 9　笑いは最高の妙薬

「笑う門には福来たる」という表現があります。「健康」でいることは「福」の基本です。
「笑う」ことはたいへん「健康」にいいということをご存知でしたか？　大いに笑って健康を保ち、幸せになりましょう。

CD Track 10

India's Giggling Guru Counsels Laughing Yourself to Good Health

Vocabulary Check（英文を読む前に意味を確認しましょう。）

- guru：教祖　　- giggle：クスクス笑う　　- multinational：多国籍企業
- Hewlett-Packard Co.：（米）コンピューター、計測機器の大手メーカ
- Volvo：スウェーデンを本拠とする自動車製造会社　　- Bangalore：【地名】バンガロール（インド）
- donate：寄付する　　- building contractor：建築請負業者　　- anonymous：匿名の
- tycoon：財界の大物　　- headquarters：本部　　- yoga：ヨガ　　- envision：将来のことを想像する
- alternative medicine：代替医療　　- endorphin：エンドルフィン、幸福ホルモン
- towering：影響力などが大きい　　- bald：はげた　　- testify：証明する　　- U. S. Senate：米国上院
- qualified doctor：有資格医師　　- medical literature：医学文献　　- stress-buster：ストレス解消（法）
- field-test：実地に試験する　　- hyena：【動物】ハイエナ　　- swell：（数が）増える
- recount：話す　　- gag：ギャグ、ジョーク　　- fake：偽りの　　- digestion：消化
- nonprofit：非営利の　　- reap：得る　　- abdominal：腹部の　　- trigger：引き起こす

・自信のある人は英文をできるだけ速く読み、時間を計ってください。苦手な人はゆっくり読みましょう。

　India's "guru of giggling," Madan Kataria — who travels constantly spreading his "laugh with no reason" gospel — has been hired by multinationals from computer giant Hewlett-Packard to automaker Volvo to hold team-building laughter sessions. Now he is setting up a "laughter university" in the southern city of Bangalore on land donated by a building contractor and $250,000 from an anonymous tycoon. "In three months we will start building and by the end of 2013 we will be up and running. We want to build a worldwide community headquarters of laughter yoga," he said.

　Kataria envisions holding laughter sessions and conferences at the center and setting up an alternative medicine unit to expand medical knowledge about the beneficial health effects of laughter. Studies already suggest laughter releases feel-good endorphins, the brain chemicals that are linked with a sense of well-being. "Laughing is the healthiest thing you can do — it's the best medicine," said the towering, bald 58-year-old, whose movement has inspired thousands of "laughter clubs" in India and around the world from Beirut to Dublin. Kataria also holds laughter sessions in schools, prisons, hospitals and retirement homes, and a few years ago testified before a U.S. Senate committee that laughter yoga could help the country cut health care costs.

A qualified doctor, he hit upon medical literature advocating laughter as a stress-buster and remedy for other ailments. In 1995, he decided to field-test his findings before setting up the first of his clubs. Kataria started with four strangers in a Mumbai park. They stood in a circle and "laughed like hyenas," he recalled. Their number soon swelled to around 50. They recounted jokes but realized they didn't have enough gags — then Kataria found the body was unable to distinguish between fake and genuine laughter with both producing the same "happy, healing chemistry." "Anyway, fake laughter turns into real laughter after a few moments. Try it," he advised. He persuaded his group to laugh with him for one minute with no reason. It stretched into 10 minutes as the laughter turned infectious, and the Laughter Yoga movement was born.

　"Laughter is more about social connection and bonding than something being funny," said Amit Sood, a doctor at the Mayo Clinic in the United States. "Studies show all kinds of benefits from laughter from better immunity and coping skills, lower stress, better relationships to improved digestion."

　Kataria, who runs his nonprofit Laughter Yoga Institute with a dozen employees from his Mumbai home, says one needs a full 15 to 20 minutes of giggling daily to reap the full benefits. Researchers believe it may be the use of abdominal muscles in laughing that triggers the release of endorphins — a phenomenon also associated with physical exercise. "It's not enough to just watch a funny movie since you just laugh a few seconds at a funny line — you need to laugh for a stretch to get the rewards," Kataria said.

(484 words)

(The Japan Times, Nov. 30, 2012)

(AFP-JIJI)

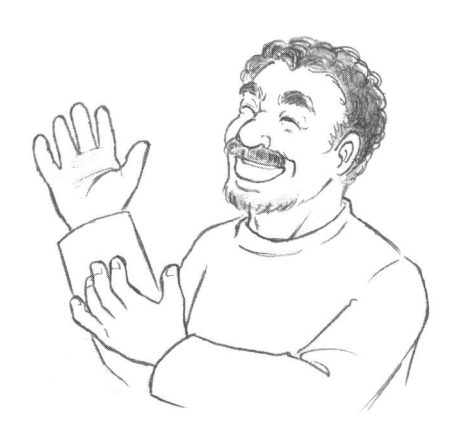

速読をした人は wpm を確認しましょう。

計算式：（あなたのwpm）＝総単語数（484）／（かかった時間（分））　　　あなたのwpm：　　　　　　wpm

（参考）	2分	242wpm	2.5分	194wpm	3分	161wpm
	3.5分	138wpm	4分	121wpm	4.5分	108wpm
	5分	97wpm	5.5分	88wpm		

内容把握問題　次の１～５の英文が、本文の内容と一致する場合はT、一致しない場合はFを（　）内に記入しましょう。

1. (　) American multinationals are not interested in the beneficial effects of laughter.
2. (　) Kataria doesn't think that laughter yoga can cut health care costs.
3. (　) The human body is able to distinguish between fake and genuine laughter.
4. (　) Kataria doesn't believe it is enough to laugh for just a few seconds to trigger the release of endorphins.
5. (　) Studies show many kinds of benefits from laughter, such as better immunity and lower stress.

上記の問題はいくつできましたか？　正解率をあなたのwpm の値にかけてみましょう。

計算式：（あなたの読解効率）＝（あなたのwpm）×（（正答数）／ 5）　　　あなたの読解効率：

語句問題　本文中に出てくる次の１～５の語句とほぼ同じ意味を表すものをa～dの中から１つ選びましょう。

1. conference
   a. luggage　　　b. meeting　　　c. trial　　　d. party
2. well-being
   a. loneliness　　b. anger　　　c. sadness　　　d. happiness
3. ailment
   a. cold　　　b. illness　　　c. stomachache　　　d. depression
4. stretch
   a. shorten　　　b. withdraw　　　c. lie　　　d. prolong
5. benefit
   a. advantage　　b. disadvantage　　c. present　　　d. medicine

文法解説【受動態】

本文では次の例で受動態を使い、「Madan Kataria 氏」の立場から、「多国籍企業」に行為を受けたという関係を表しています。これを能動態にすると、「多国籍企業」の立場から、目的語の「Madan Kataria 氏」に行為を行うという関係を表します。

India's "guru of giggling," Madan Kataria has been hired by multinationals.【受動態】
 (= Multinationals have hired India's "guru of giggling," Madan Kataria.【能動態】)

① 受動態のつくり方

Laughter releases endorphins.（能動態）
→ ① Endorphins ② are released ③ by laughter.（受動態）
(1) 能動態の文の目的語 'endorphins' を受動態の主語にする。
(2) 能動態の動詞の時制をもとに、be + 過去分詞の形にする。　　'are released'
(3) 能動態の文の主語を受動態では by + 目的格にする。　　'by laughter'

② 時制による形

現在形	Laughter releases endorphins.	→ Endorphins are released by laughter.
過去形	Laughter released endorphins.	→ Endorphins were released by laughter.
未来形	Laughter will release endorphins.	→ Endorphins will be released by laughter.
現在完了形	Laughter has released endorphins.	→ Endorphins have been released by laughter.
過去完了形	Laughter had released endorphins.	→ Endorphins had been released by laughter.
未来完了形	Laugher will have released endorphins.	→ Endorphins will have been released by laughter.
現在進行形	Laugher is releasing endorphins.	→ Endorphins are being released by laughter.
過去進行形	Laugher was releasing endorphins.	→ Endorphins were being released by laughter.

【参考】
※第4文型の受動態 ⇒第4文型では目的語が2つあるので、2種類の受動態ができます。
【例】She showed me the way.
→ a) I was shown the way by her. / b) The way was shown to me by her.
 b) の間接目的語 me の前には、ふつう to もしくは for をおきます。

※ by ～ の省略

by us, by you, by them のような動作主が一般的な人をさす場合、動作主が不明な場合は by + 動作主はしばしば省略されます。
　　Many children were killed in the accident.

※句動詞の受動態

take care of ～「～の世話をする」のような熟語（句動詞）の場合は、能動文の句動詞のあとの目的語が受動態の主語となります。
【例】I took care of my brother. → My brother was taken care of by me.

文法問題 次の1〜6の英文を受動態の文に、7〜10の英文を能動態の文になおしましょう。

1. Every patient respects the doctor.
2. The nurse showed me the way to the waiting room.（2通りの受動態の文に）
3. He is taking the medicine.
4. The doctor gave him an injection.（2通りの受動態の文に）
5. His movement has inspired thousands of "laughter clubs."
6. Kataria holds laughter sessions.
7. She will be helped by laughter yoga.
8. Many patients are made happy by the doctor.
9. He had to be persuaded to laugh.
10. Malaria is caused by the bite of an infected mosquito.

英作文 次の1〜5の日本文を英語になおしましょう。

1. 彼は妻の笑顔（smile）に救われた。
2. 母は3人の医者に治療を受けた（treat）。
3. 疲れた魂（tired soul）は音楽によって癒される（heal）。
4. アロマセラピー（aromatherapy）が患者の緊張（tension）を和らげる（reduce）ために使われている。
5. 私のお気に入りのハーブティー（favorite herbal tea）がコンビニで売られている。

Let's think!

今までどのような場面で「笑った」のかを思い出して、自分にとって何が「笑いの種」となるのかをまとめてみましょう。

Let's make a speech!

「笑い」が自分や周りの人々の気持ちとその場の雰囲気を変えたエピソードを思い出し、「笑い」の大切さについて、英語で3分間のスピーチをしてみましょう。

Column ① 「統合医療」(Integrative Medicine)

「統合医療」とは、西洋医学による医療と代替医療をあわせた治療のことです。統合医療は、西洋医学に代替医療を加えることによって、病気の早期発見や予防、健康維持なども目指しています。

「代替医療」は、ハーブ療法、マッサージ療法、音楽療法、リフレクソロジー、瞑想療法、イメージ療法、芸術療法、タッチ療法等があり、WHOによれば医学的論拠が認められる代替医療は世界に約100あるといいます。本文に出てきた「笑い」(ユーモア)もこの1つで、これらは西洋医療に比べて副作用が少ないことが特徴です。日本では漢方などを除き大半は保険適用外ですが、西洋医療を補う治療法として注目されています。

「統合医療」という言葉の最初の発案者は、Andrew Weil博士(米国の健康医学研究者、医学博士)で、人間に本来備わっている自然治癒力を引き出す統合医療を提唱している人物です。統合医療を診療で実践できる医師を育成するための教育プログラム(統合医療プログラム)を、米アリゾナ大学医学部で行っています。著書 *Spontaneous Healing*(日本語訳:『癒す心、治る力』)と *Eating Well for Optimum Health*(日本語訳:『アンドルー・ワイル博士の医食同源』)は米国でベストセラーとなりました。

アリゾナ大学統合医療プログラムを修了した9名の日本人医師が中心となって「統合医療」についての『統合医療とは何か？が、わかる本』(ほんの木、2012)も出版されています。

日本においては、日本統合医療学会、日本補完代替医療学会などが中心になり、統合医療の実現のための教育、研究などを進めています。

Column ② 映画 *Patch Adams*

1998年の米国映画 *Patch Adams*(邦題『パッチ・アダムス・トゥルー・ストーリー』)は、「ユーモアこそが最良の薬」という考えを実践し、医療とは何かを問い続けた実在の医師をモデルにした感動のヒューマンドラマです。ロビン・ウィリアムズ(Robin Williams)が、医学界の常識を覆した医学生パッチ・アダムスに扮しています。自殺癖を持つアダムスは、自らの意志で心療内科に入院し、そこで「笑い」が心の癒しになると気づき、医学の道を志します。2年後、ヴァージニア大学の医学部に入学し、患者をユーモアで楽しませていました。しかし、彼の考えは、学部長や仲間に理解されませんでした。そこで彼は自分の信念を貫くために恋人とともに無料治療院を開設します。

ぜひご覧いただきたい作品です。

Chapter 10　iPSは人類の夢

京都大学の山中伸也教授がiPS細胞を発見し、ノーベル賞を受賞しました。
iPS細胞は世界中の病に苦しむ人たちが待ち望んだ朗報です。

CD Track 11

World's First Clinical Trials with Human iPS Cells OK'd

Vocabulary Check（英文を読む前に意味を確認しましょう。）

- clinical trial：臨床試験
- induced pluripotent stem (iPS) cell：人工（誘導）多能性幹細胞、iPS 細胞
- harvest：採取する
- age-related：加齢に関連した
- macular degeneration：黄斑変性（症）
- presently：現在
- untreatable：治療不可能な
- Riken Center for Developmental Biology：理化学研究所、発生・再生科学総合研究センター
- Foundation for Biomedical Research and Innovation：公益財団法人 先端医療振興財団
- retinal：網膜の
- transplant：移植する、移植
- incurable：不治の
- groundbreaking：画期的な
- embryo：（人間の）胎芽、胚（受精卵が分裂を始めてから8週目の終わりまでの、分化が終了する前の状態をさす）
- embryonic：胚の
- crucially：重要なことに
- physiology：生理学
- tissue：（細胞の）組織

・自信のある人は英文をできるだけ速く読み、時間を計ってください。苦手な人はゆっくり読みましょう。

　The government has signed off on the world's first clinical trials to use induced pluripotent stem (iPS) cells harvested from the bodies of human patients. Health minister Norihisa Tamura on Friday gave his seal of approval to a proposal by two research institutes that will allow them to begin tests aimed at treating age-related macular degeneration, a common medical condition that causes blindness in older people, using iPS cells. The pioneering field of stem-cell research may one day offer cures for conditions that are presently untreatable, and scientists hope these macular degeneration clinical trials could offer hope to millions of people robbed of their sight.

　A government committee last month approved proposals for the tests, which will be jointly conducted by the Riken Center for Developmental Biology and the Foundation for Biomedical Research and Innovation, both in Kobe. Riken will harvest stem cells using skin cells taken from patients, a spokesman said. The trial treatment will attempt to create retinal cells that can be transplanted into six patients, replacing the damaged part of the eye. The transplants may be conducted as early as the middle of next year at the foundation's hospital, he said. Age-related macular degeneration, a condition that is incurable at present, affects mostly middle-aged and older people and can lead to blindness. Approximately 700,000 people in Japan alone have the condition.

Stem cells are infant cells that can develop into any part of the body. Until the groundbreaking discovery of iPS cells by Shinya Yamanaka of Kyoto University in 2006, the only way to obtain stem cells was to harvest them from human embryos. This is controversial because it requires the destruction of the embryo, a process that religious conservatives, among others, oppose. Like embryonic stem cells, iPS cells are also capable of developing into any cell in the body, but, crucially, their source material is readily available. Yamanaka was jointly awarded the Nobel prize in physiology or medicine last year for his successful generation of stem cells from adult skin tissue in 2006.

(337 words)
(The Japan Times, July 20, 2013)
(AFP-JIJI)

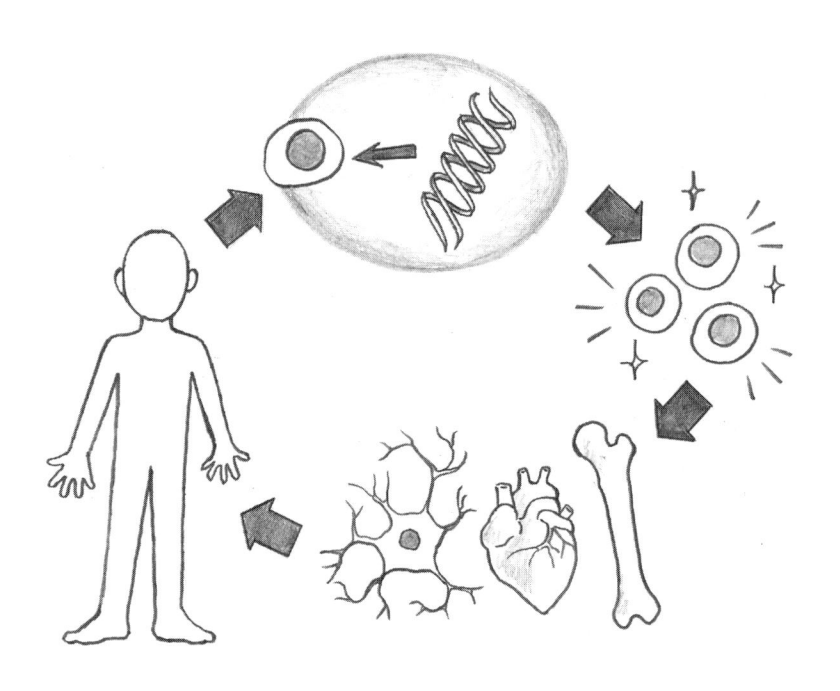

速読をした人は wpm を確認しましょう。

計算式：（あなたの wpm）＝総単語数(337) /（かかった時間(分)）　　　あなたの wpm：　　　　　　wpm

（参考）　1.5 分　225wpm　　　　2 分　169wpm　　　　2.5 分　135wpm
　　　　3 分　112wpm　　　　3.5 分　96wpm　　　　4 分　84wpm

内容把握問題　次の 1 〜 5 の英文が、本文の内容と一致する場合は T、一致しない場合は F を（　）内に記入しましょう。

1. (　) The Riken Center for Developmental Biology allowed researchers to begin tests aimed at treating age-related macular degeneration.
2. (　) The Foundation for Biomedical Research and Innovation is located in Kobe.
3. (　) Age-related macular degeneration is currently an untreatable disease.
4. (　) Transplantations of retinal cells into six patients had been conducted by 2006.
5. (　) Embryonic stem cells are capable of developing into any cell in the body.

上記の問題はいくつできましたか？　正解率をあなたの wpm の値にかけてみましょう。

計算式：（あなたの読解効率）＝（あなたの wpm）×（（正答数）/ 5）　　　あなたの読解効率：

語句問題　本文中に出てくる次の 1 〜 5 の語句とほぼ同じ意味を表すものを a 〜 d の中から 1 つ選びましょう。

1. approve
    a. refuse　　　　b. accept　　　　c. solve　　　　d. disagree
2. approximately
    a. more than　　b. less than　　　c. exactly　　　d. about
3. develop
    a. grow　　　　b. improve　　　　c. gain　　　　d. stay
4. obtain
    a. steal　　　　b. avoid　　　　c. exchange　　　d. get
5. controversial
    a. having a lot of proposal　　　　b. having a lot of violence
    c. causing a lot of disagreement　　d. causing a lot of agreement

文法解説【仮定法】

① **仮定法過去**　（「もし今、〜ならば、…するだろうに」 ⇒ 現在のことを仮定する場合）
　If + S + 動詞の過去形, S + 助動詞の過去形（would, should, could, might）+ 動詞の原形
　【例】If I were a scientist, I would try the experiment.

② **仮定法過去完了**　（「もしあの時、〜だったならば、…しただろうに」 ⇒ 過去のことを仮定する場合）
　If + S + had + 過去分詞, S + 助動詞の過去形（would, should, could, might）+ have + 過去分詞
　【例】If I had been a scientist at that time, I would have tried the experiment.

③ **未来のことを表す仮定法**
　⑴　If + S + were to + 動詞の原形, S + 助動詞の過去形 + 動詞の原形
　※まったく実現不可能な仮定から、実現の可能性のある仮定まで、さまざまな段階の仮定を表します。
　【例】If things were to be done twice, all would be wise.

　⑵　If + S + should + 動詞の原形, S + 助動詞の過去形 + 動詞の原形
　※起こる可能性が低いことを仮定する場合に用います。
　※S + 助動詞の過去形 + 動詞の原形という形以外にも、助動詞の過去形の代わりに現在形の助動詞を用いたり、命令文がくる場合があります。
　【例】If I should have macular degeneration, I will have transplantation.

④ **仮定法のさまざまな用法**
　⑴　S + wish + 過去 / 過去完了　⇒　願望を示す時に用いる
　【例】I wish I knew a good doctor.
　　　　I wish I had known a good doctor.

　⑵　as if + 過去 / 過去完了「まるで〜であるか / あったかのように」
　【例】She acts as if she were a different person at parties.
　　　　She acted as if she had been a different person at parties.

　⑶　if を用いない仮定法
　【例】Without the doctor's advice, my father would not have lived much longer.
　　　　But for the medicine, my grandmother could not go out.

文法問題 日本語を参考に、次の1〜10の英文の（　）内に適語を入れましょう。

1. 頭痛がしなければ、パーティーに出席することができるのに。
   If I (　　　) (　　　) a headache, I could attend the party.
2. あの時、その女医に出会っていなければ、私は死んでいたかもしれない。
   If I (　　　) (　　　) (　　　) the woman doctor, I might have died.
3. 彼はまるで、石で頭をぶつけた（get hit）かのようにみえる。
   He seems as if he (　　　) (　　　) on the head by a stone.
4. もしあの時、彼女があんなにお酒を飲まなかったら、今こんなに具合は悪くないだろう。
   If she (　　　) not (　　　) so much alcohol, she would (　　　) (　　　) sick.
5. 彼がもっと健康に気を配っていたら、病気にはならなかっただろうに。
   If he (　　　) (　　　) more careful about his health, he would have never got sick.
6. 医者が彼女にはっきりと説明すれば、彼女は自分の病気のことを理解できるだろうに。
   If the doctor (　　　) the condition to her clearly, she would understand her illness.
7. 彼女はいまにも気絶しそうだ。
   She looks as if she (　　　) about to faint.
8. 去年健康診断を受けていたらなあ。
   I wish I (　　　) (　　　) a checkup last year.
9. 私が今具合が悪いかのように、私に話しかけないで。
   Don't talk to me as if I (　　　) sick now!
10. 今退院できればなあ。
    I wish I (　　　) (　　　) the hospital now.

英作文 次の1〜5の日本文を仮定法を用いて英語になおしましょう。
1. 私が医師だったらいいのに。
2. その患者さんは子供のようにふるまう（behave）。
3. iPS細胞がもっと早く発見されていたら（be discovered earlier）、彼は助かっていたかもしれなかったのに。
4. もし（今）、政府が臨床試験（clinical test）を承認（approve）すれば、研究者たちはすぐに研究を始めることができるのに。
5. 日本政府が（あの時）若い研究者を支援していたら、彼はノーベル賞を受賞できて（receive the Nobel Prize）いたかもしれないのに。

Let's think!

iPS細胞は夢の細胞といわれていますが、iPS細胞によって将来どのようなことが期待できるのかを調べてみましょう。

Let's make a speech!

人類を多くの苦しみから救うことができるiPS細胞ですが、iPS細胞の利点だけでなく、問題点も考え、光と影の部分両方をもりこんで英語で3分間のスピーチをしてみましょう。

Chapter 10 iPSは人類の夢

> **Column**
> [コラム]
>
> ## iPS 細胞
>
> iPS（induced pluripotent stem cell）細胞は 2006 年に京都大学の山中伸弥教授（2012 年にノーベル医学生理学賞を受賞）のグループによってつくり出された人工多能性幹細胞です。人間の皮膚などの体細胞に、ごく少数の因子を導入し、培養することによって、さまざまな組織や臓器の細胞に分化する能力とほぼ無限に増殖する能力をもつ多能性幹細胞に変化します。病気の原因の解明、新しい薬の開発、細胞移植治療などに無現の可能性を持っています。
>
> 世界初の iPS 細胞に特化した先駆的な中核研究機関としての役割を果たすため、京都大学iPS 細胞研究所（Center for iPS Cell Research and Application, Kyoto University、略称：CiRA（サイラ））が、2010 年 4 月 1 日設立されました。27 の研究グループが iPS 細胞に関する情報やアイディアなどを共有して日夜研究に励んでいます。
>
> iPS 研究は、今や世界で競争が繰り広げられ、さまざまな成果がでています。例えば 2014 年 5 月には、アカゲザルに自分の iPS 細胞から成長させた骨髄細胞を移植し、腫瘍をつくらずに体内で骨を再生させることに成功したと、米国立衛生研究所（NIH）のチームが米科学誌セル・リポーツに発表しています。
>
> 日本は今まで以上に国際競争力を身に付ける必要に迫られています。国際競争力をつけ、国内で最先端の医療を行うだけでなく、国際貢献をすることが世界から求められているのです。

Chapter 11 薬のネット販売に一定のルールを

インターネットショッピングは私たちの生活を便利なものにしてくれます。2013年には、ほぼすべての市販薬がインターネットで販売できるようになりました。市販薬のオンライン販売について、利点とリスクを考えてみましょう。

CD Track 12

Rules for Online Drug Sales

Vocabulary Check（英文を読む前に意味を確認しましょう。）

- the revised Pharmaceutical Affairs Law：改正薬事法　● go into force：発効する
- the Health and Welfare Ministry：厚生労働省　● ordinance：法令
- nonprescription drug：非処方薬（市販薬）[over-the-counter drug (OTC)「対面販売薬」ともいう]
- side effect：副作用　● pharmacist：薬剤師
- the Supreme Court's Second Petit Bench：最高裁第二法廷
- null and void：無意味で法的に無効である　● hair tonic：ヘアトニック
- mobility：機動性、移動性　● heed：留意する　● legally：法的に、法律上
- unreasonable：非現実的な、不合理な　● liberalize：～を自由化する
- misleading：誤解を招きかねない

・自信のある人は英文をできるだけ速く読み、時間を計ってください。苦手な人はゆっくり読みましょう。

　In June 2009, when the revised Pharmaceutical Affairs Law went into force, the Health and Welfare Ministry issued an ordinance dividing nonprescription drugs into three categories in accordance with the intensity of their possible side effects. Drugs of the first category were to be sold only by pharmacists while drugs of the second and third categories could be sold by either pharmacists or registered drug sellers. Only nonprescription drugs in the third category, such as vitamins, were allowed to be sold online.

　On Jan. 11, 2013, the Supreme Court's Second Petit Bench ruled 4-0 that the Health and Welfare Ministry's ban on the sale of nonprescription drugs over the Internet is null and void. Since the ruling, some mail order companies have started vigorously selling such drugs over the Internet, including drugs whose sale over the Internet had been prohibited. Such sales will likely expand in the absence of rules to regulate them. Some companies have even started selling hair tonics that could cause health problems for people with heart disease. Certain rules are clearly necessary. For example, consumers should be strongly urged to read drug instructions, including warnings of possible side effects, prior to use of the product.

　Online sales are convenient for people who are too busy, have mobility problems or live in remote areas. But convenience should not take priority over safety. Associations of patients and consumers point out that expert warnings are necessary not only about the risks of nonprescription drugs themselves but also about the risks of combined use of prescription and nonprescription drugs. The government should heed their concerns. It will be difficult to legally restrict the sale of nonprescription drugs over the Internet. The Health and Welfare Ministry has set up a panel to work out rules for such sales together with consumers, patients and mail-order firms.

 It would be unreasonable to completely liberalize the sale of nonprescription drugs over the Internet in the absence of a system that will ensure that consumers fully understand the correct use of drugs and the measures that they should take when they suffer from the unwelcome side effects of drugs. But a system is needed to ban online sellers who provide misleading or false information about drugs. The ministry panel has great responsibility.

(377 words)

(The Japan Times, Mar. 15, 2013)

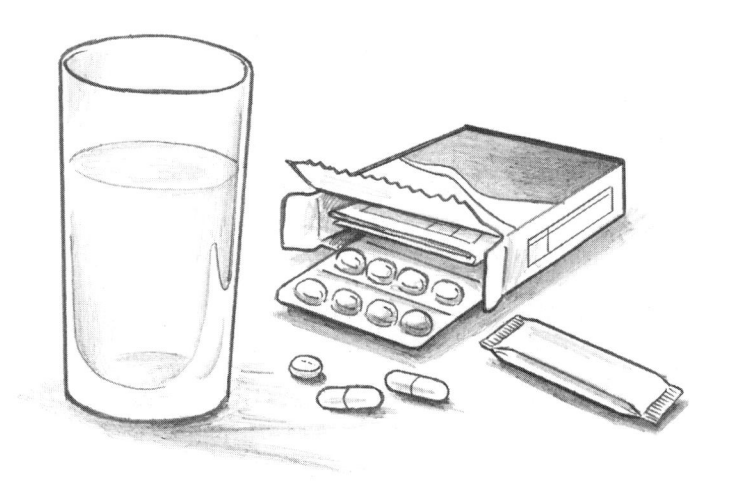

速読をした人は wpm を確認しましょう。

計算式：（あなたのwpm）＝総単語数(377)/(かかった時間(分))　　　あなたのwpm：　　　　　wpm

（参考）　1.5分　251wpm　　　2分　189wpm　　　2.5分　151wpm
　　　　 3分　126wpm　　　3.5分　108wpm　　　4分　94wpm
　　　　 4.5分　84wpm　　　5分　75wpm

内容把握問題　次の1～5の英文が、本文の内容と一致する場合はT、一致しない場合はFを（　）内に記入しましょう。

1. (　　) The Japanese government decided to allow most nonprescription drugs to be sold online in June, 2009.
2. (　　) The Supreme Court ruled that the government's attempt to regulate online sales of drugs was illegal.
3. (　　) Vitamins and hair tonics are prohibited from being sold over the Internet.
4. (　　) Online sales of nonprescription drugs are considered beneficial to people who cannot buy drugs in person.
5. (　　) It is important to build a system to ensure consumer access to safe and convenient online sales of drugs.

上記の問題はいくつできましたか？　正解率をあなたのwpmの値にかけてみましょう。

計算式：（あなたの読解効率）＝（あなたのwpm）×((正答数) / 5)　　　あなたの読解効率：

語句問題　本文中に出てくる次の1～5の語句とほぼ同じ意味を表すものをa～dの中から1つ選びましょう。

1. prohibit
    a. ban　　　　　b. allow　　　　c. limit　　　　d. order
2. regulate
    a. decide　　　 b. control　　　c. consume　　　d. practice
3. convenient
    a. easy　　　　 b. cheep　　　　c. friendly　　　d. useful
4. instruction
    a. direction　　 b. lesson　　　 c. bill　　　　　d. value
5. measure
    a. scale　　　　b. degree　　　c. means　　　　d. condition

文法解説【疑問詞】

疑問詞は、「誰（who）」、「何（what）」、「どれ（which）」、「いつ（when）」、「どこで（where）」、「なぜ（why）」、「どのように（how）」など、知りたい情報を尋ねる時に用いる語で、疑問代名詞、疑問形容詞、疑問副詞があります。

① **疑問代名詞**　（「人」や「物事」について尋ねる場合）
　【疑問代名詞の種類】who, whose,（whom）, which, what
　【例】Who said such a thing?

② **疑問形容詞**　（名詞の前に置いて「誰の〜」、「何の〜」、「どちらの〜」と尋ねる場合）
　【疑問形容詞の種類】　whose, what, which
　【例】Which picture do you prefer, this or that?

③ **疑問副詞**　（「場所」、「時」、「理由」、「方法」について尋ねる場合）
　【疑問副詞の種類】　when, where, why, how
　【例】When did the earthquake happen?

④ **間接疑問**　（疑問を表す名詞節が文の一部になる場合）
　（1）疑問詞が導く場合　⇒　疑問詞 + S + V
　【例】We don't know what he wants to do.
　　　　（= We don't know ＋ What does he want to do?）
　（2）疑問詞のない関節疑問　⇒　if (whether) + S + V
　【例】The doctor did not know whether the drug had any side effect.

　　think, suppose, consider などの動詞を使って挿入的に入れる場合 ⇒ 疑問詞＋挿入句＋ S + V
　　　What do you think the child needs?
　　　When do you suppose he will wake up?

⑤ **疑問詞＋ to 不定詞**　（what, which, where, when, how などの疑問詞のあとに、to 不定詞がつく場合）
　【例】It is important to consider how to achieve convenient and safe drug purchases.

文法問題 日本語を参考に、次の1〜10の英文の（　）内に適語を入れましょう。

1. どうしてそんなにひどい事故が起こったの？
   (   ) caused such a terrible accident?
2. ここから病院までの距離を教えてくれませんか。
   Could you tell me (   ) far it is from here to the hospital?
3. 深刻な薬の副作用が生じた時の対処法が分からない。
   I don't know (   ) to do when I suffer the severe side effects of drugs.
4. 多くの人は、その薬が安全かどうかを知りたがっている。
   Many people want to know (   ) the medicine is safe.
5. 今までにどのような治療をしましたか。
   (   ) treatment have you tried?
6. 夜中に何回トイレに起きますか。
   (   ) (   ) times do you get up at night to urinate?
7. どうすると痛みが和らぎますか。
   (   ) decreases your pain?
8. どこがかゆいですか。
   (   ) do you feel itchy?
9. 今日はどうされましたか。
   (   ) is the matter with you today?
10. これは誰の聴診器かしら。
    I wonder (   ) stethoscope this is.

英作文 次の1〜5の日本文を疑問詞を用いて英語になおしましょう。

1. インターネットでの非処方箋薬（nonprescription drugs）販売は、いつ許可された（be allowed）のですか。
2. 薬のオンライン販売（online sales）についてだれが責任を負っているのですか。
3. いつその法律が発効（go into force）されたか知っていますか。
4. その薬がどこで売られているのか教えてください。
5. その薬についての情報をどのようにして得たらいいのか分かりません。

Let's think!

インターネットショッピングの利点とリスクについて英語でまとめてみましょう。

Let's make a speech!

「薬のインターネット販売」について、賛成、反対両方の立場に分かれて英語で3分間スピーチをしてみましょう。

> **Column [コラム]　薬のインターネット販売が解禁されるまで**
>
> 　2012年、厚生労働省がまとめた「医薬品・医療機器等安全性情報」によると、2007年から2011年までの5年間に、市販薬（OTC）の副作用についての報告は1,220件あり、うち24例が死亡例でした。副作用がもっとも多かったのは、総合感冒薬（404例）、次いで解熱鎮痛消炎薬（243例）で、風邪薬や鎮痛剤などの危険度が高いといえます。死亡したケースは、総合感冒薬の12例、解熱鎮痛消炎薬の4例、漢方製剤の2例であり、後遺症となったケースは、総合感冒薬で8例、解熱鎮痛消炎薬で2例、カルシウム薬で2例報告されていました。このような背景もあって、厚労省は市販薬のインターネット販売の全面解禁については慎重な姿勢でした。しかし、2013年1月の最高裁判決を契機に、一部の解熱鎮痛剤や鼻炎用薬を除いて、市販薬約11,400品目のほとんど（99％）のネット販売が可能となりました。

Chapter 12　血液検査による出生前診断、始まる

晩婚化が進み、高齢出産が増えています。2011年には全出産件数の25％が35歳以上の妊婦によるものでした。しかしながら妊婦の年齢と共に染色体異常の確率も上がります。ダウン症の子供は、20歳の妊婦では1500人に1人の割合ですが、35歳の場合400人に1人、40歳では100人に1人となるといわれています。そんな中、2013年に新しい出生前診断技術が導入されました。記事を読んで、この問題について考えてみましょう。

CD Track 13

New Prenatal Diagnosis May Start Next Month

Vocabulary Check（英文を読む前に意味を確認しましょう。）

- prenatal diagnosis：出生前診断　● chromosomal abnormalities：染色体異常　● fetus：胎児
- The Japan Society of Obstetrics and Gynecology：日本産科婦人科学会
- authorize：認可する、公認する
- the Japanese Association of Medical Sciences：日本医学会　● utilize：利用する
- authorization：認可　● amniotic fluid check：羊水検査　● inject：注射する　● belly：腹部
- miscarriage：流産　● maternal serum screenings：母体血清マーカー検査
- the Japan Society for Human Genetics：日本人類遺伝学会　● embryo screening：胎児選別
- prerequisite：前提条件　● obstetrician：産科医　● pediatrician：小児科医
- specialize：専門とする　● genetics：遺伝子学　● outpatient：外来患者　● ultrasound：超音波
- eligible：適格な

・自信のある人は英文をできるだけ速く読み、時間を計ってください。苦手な人はゆっくり読みましょう。

　A new method of prenatal diagnosis that can reveal chromosomal abnormalities in a fetus merely through an analysis of the mother's blood may be adopted as early as next month at a limited number of institutions, the Japan Society of Obstetrics and Gynecology has said. Institutions authorized by the Japanese Association of Medical Sciences to utilize the new method must meet certain requirements, and all cases should be treated as clinical trials, according to the guidelines announced Saturday. Applications for authorization can be submitted beginning this week.

　The new test examines fetuses' DNA using a sample of their mothers' blood. Unlike the standard amniotic fluid check, in which a needle must be injected into a pregnant woman's belly, there is no chance it will cause a miscarriage. The new prenatal diagnosis method is also more accurate than maternal serum screenings in determining whether fetuses have chromosomal abnormalities. The serum test, also a blood test, can only give the probability of such problems occurring.

　If results from the latest method are negative, meaning the fetus shows no signs of chromosomal abnormalities, the chance of the fetus being born without such abnormalities is greater than 99 percent. However, if the test turns out positive, the rate of accuracy can differ considerably depending on the age of the mother, and therefore an amniotic fluid check is required to identify chromosomal abnormalities.

The Japan Society of Obstetrics and Gynecology announced the latest guidelines at a press conference in Tokyo along with the Japanese Association of Medical Sciences, the Japan Society for Human Genetics and other related parties. The organizations issued a joint statement calling for careful introduction of the new method, acknowledging concerns it could promote "embryo screening."

According to the guidelines, institutions wishing to become authorized to carry out the new prenatal diagnosis test should meet prerequisites such as:

■ Having full-time obstetricians and pediatricians on staff.
■ Ensuring at least a few of such doctors also specialize in genetics.
■ Having an outpatient genetics department.
■ Having the ability to provide pregnant women with extensive information and genetic counseling.

Furthermore, the guidelines say the new method should only be used on women who:

■ Are carrying fetuses that may have chromosomal abnormalities, as indicated by ultrasound and other examinations.
■ Have previously become pregnant with babies showing such abnormalities.
■ Are pregnant relatively late in life.

Regarding the last point, the guidelines do not mention a specific age, although a draft version announced in December said women aged 35 or older were eligible for the new test.

(423 words)

(The Daily Yomiuri, Mar. 11, 2013)

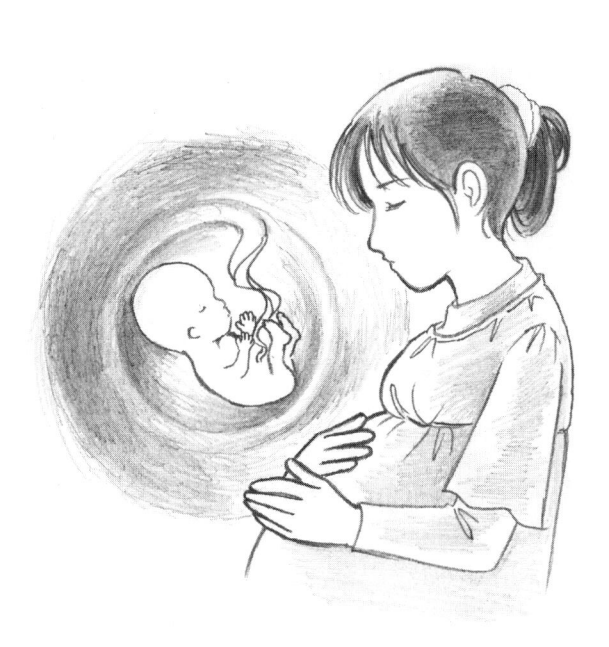

速読をした人はwpmを確認しましょう。

計算式：（あなたのwpm）＝総単語数(422)／（かかった時間(分)）　　あなたのwpm：　　　　　wpm

（参考）　2分　211wpm　　　2.5分　169wpm　　　3分　141wpm
　　　　3.5分　121wpm　　　4分　106wpm　　　4.5分　94wpm
　　　　5分　84wpm　　　　5.5分　77wpm

内容把握問題　次の1～5の英文が、本文の内容と一致する場合はT、一致しない場合はFを（　）内に記入しましょう。

1. (　) The Japan Society of Obstetrics and Gynecology has authorized hospitals to conduct the new prenatal blood test.
2. (　) The new prenatal blood test can detect chromosomal abnormalities in fetuses more accurately than maternal serum screenings.
3. (　) When the result of the new prenatal blood test is positive, it means the fetus has some abnormality.
4. (　) To conduct the prenatal blood test, institutions are required to have full-time obstetricians and pediatricians with sufficient knowledge and experience in prenatal diagnosis.
5. (　) The prenatal blood test will be available to pregnant women aged 35 or older.

上記の問題はいくつできましたか？　正解率をあなたのwpmの値にかけてみましょう。

計算式：（あなたの読解効率）＝（あなたのwpm）×（（正答数）／5）　　あなたの読解効率：

語句問題　本文中に出てくる次の1～5の語句とほぼ同じ意味を表すものをa～dの中から1つ選びましょう。

1. adopt
    a. approve　　b. release　　c. suppose　　d. apply
2. identify
    a. stimulate　　b. detect　　c. visualize　　d. record
3. probability
    a. loyalty　　b. certainty　　c. usability　　d. likelihood
4. extensive
    a. much　　b. little　　c. wrong　　d. limited
5. previously
    a. recently　　b. once　　c. formerly　　d. unexpectedly

文法解説【否定形】

英語の否定は、否定・準否定の形容詞（no, little, few など）、否定・準否定の副詞（not, never, hardly, rarely など）、否定の代名詞（nothing, nobody, none など）によって表されます。

① 名詞を否定する場合
(1) no（no ＋ 名詞）
【例（本文）】The fetus shows no signs of chromosomal abnormalities.
※ nothing, nobody, none は、〔no ＋ 名詞〕と同じ働きをします。
【例】Nobody（＝ No one）was injured in the accident.
(2) little, few（数や量が）ほとんどない
【例】There are few hospitals that perform the prenatal blood test.

② 動詞を否定する場合
(1) not（〔be 動詞 ＋ not〕、〔do / does / did ＋ not ＋ 動詞の原形〕、〔助動詞 ＋ not ＋ 動詞の原形〕）
【例（本文）】The guidelines do not mention a specific age.
(2) hardly / scarcely は「（程度が）ほとんどない」、rarely / seldom は「（頻度が）ほとんどない」
hardly, scarcely, rarely, seldom は副詞のため、not と同じ位置に置きます。
【例】The injured child could hardly walk.

③ 部分否定
否定語に always, necessarily, completely, altogether, absolutely, all, every などの「全体性」や「完全性」を表す語が続く場合、「全部が（完全に）〜というわけではない」という部分否定を表します。
【例】Rich people are not always happy.

④ 二重否定
否定を表す語が2つ重なり、肯定の意味を表すものを二重否定といいます。
【例】Such incidents are not uncommon.

⑤ 否定による倒置
否定を表す副詞（句）が文頭に置かれた場合に、倒置（疑問文の語順になること）が起きます。
【例】Little did the doctors know the complication would occur.

⑥ 否定の慣用表現
no longer 〜：もはや〜でない
too … to ＋ 動詞の原形 〜：あまりに…なので〜できない
the last … ＋ to ＋動詞の原形 〜：決して〜しない…　　　fail to ＋動詞の原形 〜：〜できない
anything but 〜、far from 〜：決して〜でない　　　neither A nor B：A も B も〜でない
not only A but (also) B：A だけでなく B も　　　not A but B：A でなく B
〔否定文〕, nor 〜：（先行する否定文を受けて）〜もまた〜ない

文法問題　次の1〜10の英文の（　）内に入れるのに最も適切な語を選びましょう。

1. The chemical (either / no / neither) increases nor decreases the number of bacteria.
2. Most people do not know what is toxic, (no / not / nor) do they know what reaction occurs.
3. There has been (not / no / nothing) scientific evidence of a benefit.
4. We generally know very (little / few / no) about why children have diarrhea.
   ※ diarrhea：下痢
5. If you simply ask patients whether they took the medicine, they will likely say (neither / few / no).
6. Alzheimer's does (not / no / none) occur naturally in the mouse.
7. Very (no / few / little) people live to be 100.
8. I could (no / few / hardly) receive special clinical training at the famous hospital.
9. He (not / nobody / no) longer has any possibility of surviving.
10. We still (fail to eradicate / fail not to eradicate / does not eradicate) cancer.

英作文　次の1〜5の日本文を英語になおしましょう。

1. その胎児（fetus）に染色体異常（chromosomal abnormality）があるという疑いはほとんどない。
2. その病院では、羊水検査（amniotic fluid check）はめったに使われない。
3. その病院には常勤の産科医（obstetrician）も小児科医（pediatrician）もいなかった。
4. すべての妊婦が出生前（prenatal）血液検査を受けるとは限らない。
5. 新しい出生前診断（prenatal diagnosis）について何の言及もなされなかった。

Let's think!

下表は、2013年時点における、新型出生前診断を巡る各国の対応を示したものです。日本に先行してこの診断を実施している海外の実施状況について英語でまとめてみましょう。

	合衆国	ドイツ	イギリス	フランス	日本
検査の実態	妊婦が自由に選択	法律で遺伝カウンセリングを義務化	民間機関で実施	合衆国の会社と提携するラボが実施予定	遺伝子カウンセリング体制のある施設で、臨床研究として実施
運用方法等について、国レベルでの議論の有無	×	○	○	×	×（日本産科婦人科学会が指針を策定）
検査費用（円）	8万円〜19万円	11万円	6万円	13万円	21万円
保険適用の有無	○	×	×	×	×
障害を理由とした中絶の合法化	△（州によって異なる）	×（事実上容認）	○	○	×（事実上容認）

（読売新聞：2013年10月30日等参照）

Let's make a speech!

出生前診断を受けることについて賛成、反対の立場に分かれて、それぞれの理由を説明し、英語で3分間スピーチをしてみましょう。

Column [コラム]　新型出生前診断：命にかかわる重い検査

　妊婦の採血によって胎児の染色体異常が高い精度で発見できる「新型出生前診断」は、2013年4月から臨床研究という形で始まりました。子宮に穿刺を行う羊水検査や、繁生絨毛膜サンプリングは流産確率があり、母体血清マーカー検査は精度に問題があったのに対し、新型検査は、精度が高く、血液採取だけでよく、妊娠10週という早い時期に検査できることなどから、注目が集まりました。

　新型検査は予想以上に急速に広がり、開始後3カ月経った段階で、全国で約1500人の妊婦が受けたことがわかっています。しかしながら、正しい理解やカウンセリング体制の整備が不十分なまま話題が先行した感は否めません。岡山大学附属病院が2013年8月に557人の妊婦を対象に行った意識調査の結果、新出生前診断について「採血して検査」という検査方法を知っていたのは75％、「陽性」だった場合確定診断には羊水検査が必要であることを理解していたのはわずか35％でした。また、実際に陽性だった場合に「羊水検査を受ける」と答えたのは74％で、「羊水検査を受けずに妊娠を続ける」が20％だったのに対し、「羊水検査を受けずに中絶する」と回答した妊婦も6％いました。その理由は「少しでも異常の可能性があるから」がもっとも多く59％でした。羊水検査まで数週間かかることから「妊娠週が進んでからでは、胎児がかわいそう、母体に負担がかかる、その間不安である」という理由も多くありました。

　岡山大学の調査でもわかるように、導入の時点では、新型出生前診断についての理解がまだ十分でなく、結果によっては、産むことに対して妊婦に大きな決断を迫ることになりかねない事態となりました。このような「命の選択に係わる重い検査」を導入する際には、妊婦に正しい情報を伝え、サポートしていけるような全体的体制を整え、倫理に関しても議論を尽くす必要があります。

Chapter 13　医療通訳で大切なことは？

近年、言葉の不自由な外国人患者に適正な医療を提供するために、医療通訳などのコミュニケーション支援に対する関心が高まってきています。国境なき通訳団に関する記事を読んで、コミュニケーションを行う上で必要な言葉と文化について考えてみましょう。

CD Track 14

The Risks of Language for Health Translators

Vocabulary Check（英文を読む前に意味を確認しましょう。）

- nongovernmental organization：民間非営利団体　- Doctors Without Borders：国境なき医師団
- Kikuyu：キクユ族　- provocative：挑発的な　- euphemism：婉曲表現　- vagina：膣
- sexual intercourse：性交　- Kiswahili：スワヒリ語（= Swahili）　- emanate：発する、生じる
- co-found：共同で設立する　- on the radar：注目されて　- medication：薬
- Maasai〔Masai〕：マサイ族（の）

・自信のある人は英文をできるだけ速く読み、時間を計ってください。苦手な人はゆっくり読みましょう。

　Translators Without Borders is an American nonprofit group. It provides language services to nongovernmental organizations such as, yes, Doctors Without Borders. The group recently trained some new translators in Nairobi in how to put health information into local languages for Kenyans.

　For health translators, finding the right words is not just about language but also culture. Muthoni Gichohi is a manager for Family Health Options Kenya, the group that organized the training. She says she has no problem expressing the names of body parts in English. But as a Kikuyu she says there are some words in her first language that may be "provocative" if she said them in public. "So I have got to really put it in another way that it is still delivering the same message, but the words will be different."

　Trainer Paul Warambo says the same issue arises with Kenya's national language. "Sometimes you are also forced to use euphemisms — use a language that is more acceptable to the people. For example, in Swahili, we will not call a body part — the vagina, for example — we will not call it by its name. We use *kitu chake* — her thing. You do not just mention it by the name, you say 'her thing.'"

　The culture of a community will largely decide how words and expressions are translated into socially acceptable language. In some cases, the way people in a culture think about an activity or object becomes the translated name for that activity or object. Paul Warambo explains how the term "sexual intercourse" is commonly translated from English into Kiswahili. "We always say, in Kiswahili, '*kutenda kitendo kibaya*' — to do something bad. So, imagine sex was associated with something bad, emanating from the African cultural context."

Whether or not a community will accept or even listen to a message is especially important in health care. Lori Thicke co-founded Translators Without Borders in 1993. She says, in general, a lot of development organizations have often overlooked the importance of language in changing health behavior. "It is true that people do not think of translation. It is absolutely not on the radar, but it is so critical if you think about it, for people to get information, whether it is how to take their medication, whether it is where to find supplies in a crisis situation."

Muthoni Gichohi and her team recently opened a health information center in a Maasai community. She learned that young Maasai cannot say certain things in the presence of elders. Also, men are usually the ones who speak at public gatherings, so people might not accept a message given by a woman.

(445 words)

(Voice of America, May. 1, 2012)

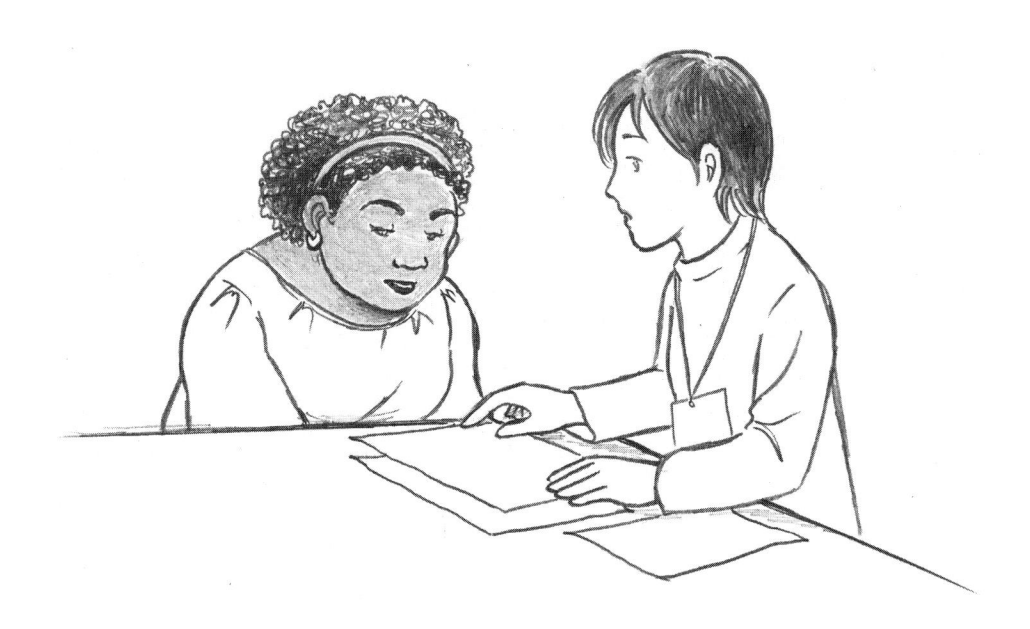

速読をした人は wpm を確認しましょう。

計算式：（あなたの wpm）＝ 445 /（かかった時間（分））　　　　あなたの wpm：　　　　　wpm

(参考)
1.5 分	297wpm	2 分	223wpm	2.5 分	178wpm
3 分	148wpm	3.5 分	127wpm	4 分	111wpm
4.5 分	99wpm	5 分	89wpm	5.5 分	81wpm

内容把握問題　次の1～5の英文が、本文の内容と一致する場合はT、一致しない場合はFを（　）内に記入しましょう。

1. (　) Translators Without Borders is a nonprofit group that sends doctors to various countries.
2. (　) Health translators need to have a good knowledge of culture as well as language.
3. (　) Translators sometimes use different words that are more acceptable to people in the community.
4. (　) The English term "sexual intercourse" is usually translated as "her thing" in Kiswahili.
5. (　) Female translators are more suitable than male ones in a Maasai community.

上記の問題はいくつできましたか？　正解率をあなたのwpmの値にかけてみましょう。

計算式：（あなたの読解効率）＝（あなたのwpm）×（（正答数）/ 5）　　　あなたの読解効率：

語句問題　本文中に出てくる次の1～5の語句とほぼ同じ意味を表すものをa～dの中から1つ選びましょう。

1. a right word
   - a. an appropriate word
   - b. an official word
   - c. a healthy word
   - d. a medical word
2. first language
   - a. standard language
   - b. dialect
   - c. words in fashion
   - d. mother tongue
3. in public
   - a. privately
   - b. in front of people
   - c. in a famous place
   - d. in a general way
4. object
   - a. focus
   - b. purpose
   - c. thing
   - d. reality
5. overlook
   - a. fail to notice
   - b. look on to
   - c. command a view of
   - d. take account of

文法解説【命令文】

命令、禁止、指示などを表すために、動詞の原形から始まる文を命令文といいます。

【命令文の種類】
① 肯定の命令文：動詞の原形 ＋ ～.
　　【例】Look at this picture.

② 否定の命令文：Don't ／ Never ＋ 動詞の原形～.
　　【例】Don't touch it.

③ 丁寧な命令文、依頼
⑴ 命令文の文頭や文末に please を加えると、やや丁寧な表現になります。
　　【例】Please open the window. / Open the window, please.

⑵ 命令文の文末に will you? を加えると、依頼を表す文となります。
　　【例】Open the window, will you?

⑶ Let's（not）＋ 動詞の原形～で提案・勧誘を表す文となります。
　　【例】Let's go out for lunch.
　　　　　Let's not talk about it now.

⑷ 指示や緊急の場合以外、助動詞を用いた方がより丁寧な表現になります。
　　【例】Please help me. ⇒ Can（Could）you help me?

④ 命令文＋, and（～しなさい、そうすれば）
　　命令文＋, or （～しなさい、そうでなければ）
　　【例】Please turn left here, and you will see a hospital.
　　　　　Please undergo surgery, or you will get much worse.

文法問題 日本文を参考に、次の1～10の英文中の（　）内に適語を入れましょう。

1. 注射の間、お子さんが動かないようにしておいてください。
   (　　　) your child still while I give her a shot.
   ※ give ～ a shot：～に注射をする
2. この書類に必要事項を記入してください。
   Please (　　　) out this form.
3. 彼の家族に至急連絡を取ってください。
   Please (　　　) some members of his family as soon as possible.
4. 体温を測りましょう。
   Let's (　　　) your temperature.
5. 血液検査の結果をご説明いたします。
   (　　　) me (　　　) the results of the blood test.
6. 「小児科はどこですか。」「2階に行って、最初の角を右に曲がってください。そうすれば、左側に見えます。」
   "Where is the Pediatrics Department?" " (　　　) upstairs and (　　　) right at the first corner. You'll find it on your left."
7. ただちにこの患者を病院の緊急治療室に運んでください。
   Please (　　　) this patient to a hospital ER at once.
   ※ ER = emergency room：緊急治療室
8. この薬を服用している時は、車を運転してはいけません。
   (　　　)(　　　) a car while you are on this medicine.
9. このベッドの上に横たわってください。
   Please (　　　) down on this bed.
10. 明日の朝は飲食をしないでください。
    (　　　)(　　　) or (　　　) anything tomorrow morning.

英作文 次の1～5の日本文を英語になおしましょう。

1. 大きく息を吸って止めてください。
2. この薬を1日に2回飲んでください。
3. お大事に。(yourself を用いて)
4. 血圧 (blood pressure) を測らせてください。(let を用いて)
5. 大丈夫ですよ。(worry を用いて)

Let's think!

世界にはどんな言語があるのか調べてみましょう。そして、もし言葉のわからない国に行くことになったらどうするか考えてみましょう。

【例】Japanese, English, Chinese, etc.

Let's make a speech!

日本や世界における医療ツーリズムの実態や課題について、参考文献やインターネットなどを調べてまとめ、英語で3分間のスピーチをしてみましょう。

Column [コラム]　医療ツーリズムと医療通訳

　インターネットの普及や国際交通網の発達によって、「医療を目的としてほかの国へ渡航する」医療ツーリズムが世界的に広がっています。現在、世界約50カ国で医療ツーリズムが実施されており、「最先端の医療技術」や「よりよい品質の医療」を求めて、年間600万人以上の医療ツーリストが国外でさまざまな検査・診療を受けています。

　日本でも、2011年に「医療滞在ビザ」を新設し、政府は医療ツーリズムを新成長戦略の一環と位置付けました。また、2013年に訪日外国人数が初めて年間1,000万人を突破しました。これらのことを背景に、厚生労働省は2014年度から、外国人の急病やけがの際の受診を手助けする「医療通訳」の育成・派遣の支援を開始しました。

　医療通訳を行うためには、一般通訳で必要な日本語および英語の言語運用能力はもちろんのこと、「問診の正確性が下がり、的確な診断・治療を施せない」「治療方針や入院に際しての注意事項などが伝えられない」といった医療の質の低下を懸念する現場の不安を解消するために、医学や薬学に関する知識、および的確な表現力も必要です。さらに、本文内で述べられていたように、患者の宗教・習慣に対する文化的知識も考慮しなければなりません。

　医療通訳士協議会（事務局・大阪大）によると、医療通訳は全国で2000人を超えますが、都市部に集中し、地方都市では少ないといいます。そのため、語学ができる医師が不在の場合、外国語に対応できないという理由で医療機関に救急搬送を断られるという場合もあるようです。

　2020年に開催される東京五輪・パラリンピックに向け、旅行者はさらに増えると見込まれています。そのため、外国人が日本で安心して医療を受けられる体制づくりが現在急ピッチで進められています。

Chapter 14 世界の子どもたちの現状を知ろう！

世界中では、今も水や衛生上の問題などで多くの子どもたちが5歳の誕生日を迎える前に亡くなっています。ユニセフなどより発表された調査報告を読んで、将来を担う世界の子どもたちの命を救う方法について考えてみましょう。

CD Track 15

Fewer Children under Age 5 Are Dying

Vocabulary Check（英文を読む前に意味を確認しましょう。）

- mortality (rate)：死亡率　● the United Nations Children's Fund：ユニセフ、国連児童基金
- the World Health Organization：世界保健機関　● the World Bank：世界銀行
- the U.N. Population Division：国連人口局　● collaborate on ～：～を共同で行う
- the World Health Organization Health Statistics and Informatics：世界保健機関保健統計情報局
- Millennium Development Goal：ミレニアム開発目標　● radically：急進的に、根本的に
- accelerate：加速する　● sub-Saharan：サハラ以南の
- the Democratic Republic of Congo：コンゴ民主共和国　● pneumonia：肺炎
- preterm birth complications：早産による合併症　● diarrhea：下痢　● obstetric：産科の
- exclusive breastfeeding：完全母乳の育児　● hygienic：衛生的な　●（umbilical）cord：臍帯

・自信のある人は英文をできるだけ速く読み、時間を計ってください。苦手な人はゆっくり読みましょう。

　A new report finds that in the past two decades, rapid progress has been made in reducing deaths among children under age five. It also says that an estimated 6.9 million children died before their fifth birthday, compared to around 12 million in 1990. Child mortality rates have fallen in all regions of the world in the past two decades, according to a new report. It says the number of deaths is down by at least 50 percent in eastern, western and southeastern Asia, as well as in northern Africa, Latin America and the Caribbean.

　The United Nations Children's Fund, the World Health Organization, the World Bank and the U.N. Population Division collaborated on the report. Ties Boerma is the chief of the World Health Organization Health Statistics and Informatics. Boerma says in the past 10 years, global child mortality has fallen by an average of more than 3 percent a year. He calls this important progress.

　But, Boerma notes it is not good enough to meet the Millennium Development Goal target of cutting child mortality by two-thirds by 2015. He says this needs to be radically accelerated to a more than 14 percent reduction in each of the next three years. "Sub-Saharan Africa and southern Asia face the greatest challenges in child survival. More than 80 percent of child deaths in the world occur in these two regions. About half of child deaths occur in just five countries — India, which actually takes 24 percent of the global total; Nigeria, 11 percent; the Democratic Republic of Congo, 7 percent; Pakistan, 5 percent and China, 4 percent of under-five deaths in the world," Boerma said. He (also) says in developed countries, one child in 152 dies before his or her fifth birthday. In Sub-Saharan Africa, he says one out of nine children dies, and in Asia that figure is one in 16. The report says globally, the leading causes of death among children under 5 are pneumonia, preterm birth complications, diarrhea, complications during birth, and malaria.

Tessa Wardlaw, the chief of monitoring and statistics for the U.N. Children's Fund, says she is encouraged by the progress being made in Sub-Saharan Africa. The region has the highest under-five mortality rate in the world, but she says the rate of decline in child deaths has more than doubled in Africa. "We welcome the widespread progress in child survival, but we importantly want to stress that there is a lot of work that remains to be done. There is unfinished business and the fact is that today on average, some 19,000 children are still dying every day from largely preventable causes," Wardlaw said.

The World Health Organization says the key to tackling these problems is to make sure women have access to health services so complications can be avoided or treated when identified. It says having emergency obstetric services at the time of delivery can save both the mother's and baby's lives. WHO also recommends home visits in the days immediately after birth to teach new mothers about the beneficial effects of exclusive breastfeeding. It says visiting nurses also can ensure proper hygienic care of the cord, and prevent women from getting infections and passing these on to their babies.

(536 words)

(Voice of America, Sep. 12, 2012)

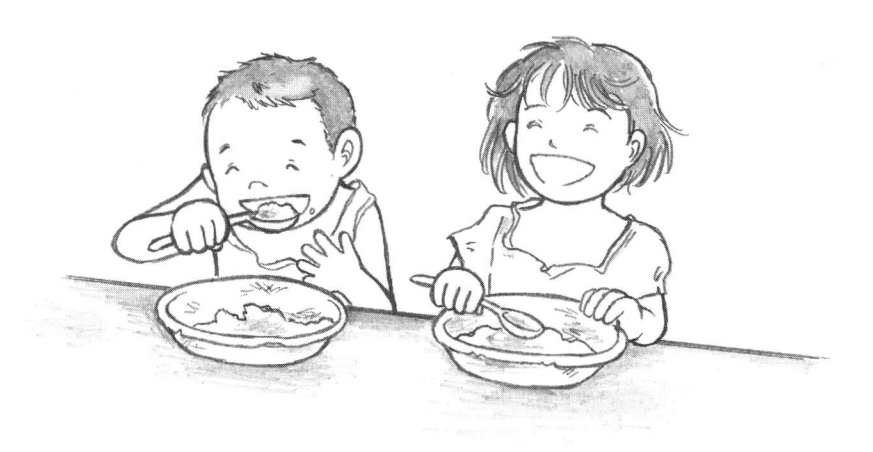

速読をした人は wpm を確認しましょう。

計算式：（あなたの wpm）＝ 536 /（かかった時間（分））　　　あなたの wpm：　　　　　wpm

(参考)	2分	268wpm	2.5分	214wpm	3分	179wpm
	3.5分	153wpm	4分	134wpm	4.5分	119wpm
	5分	107wpm	5.5分	97wpm	6分	89wpm

内容把握問題　次の1〜5の英文が、本文の内容と一致する場合は T、一致しない場合は F を（　）内に記入しましょう。

1. (　) Almost twice as many children under age five died in 2012 than in 1990.
2. (　) The Millennium Development Goal's objective is to cut child mortality by two-thirds by 2015.
3. (　) India has the highest percentage of child deaths in the world.
4. (　) Malaria and diarrhea are among the leading causes of death for children under five.
5. (　) According to the WHO, the system of home visits is not effective in preventing new mothers from getting infectious diseases.

上記の問題はいくつできましたか？　正解率をあなたの wpm の値にかけてみましょう。

計算式：（あなたの読解効率）＝（あなたの wpm）×（（正答数）/ 5）　　　あなたの読解効率：

語句問題　本文中に出てくる次の1〜5の語句とほぼ同じ意味を表すものを a〜d の中から1つ選びましょう。

1. at least
    a. not more than　　b. not less than　　c. no more than　　d. no less than
2. a challenge
    a. an active participation　　　b. a disagreement
    c. a good chance　　　　　　　d. a difficult task
3. leading
    a. worst　　b. major　　c. pacesetting　　d. terrible
4. delivery
    a. manner of speaking　　　b. distribution
    c. childbirth　　　　　　　　d. shipment
5. pass A on to B
    a. infect B with A　　b. spend A with B　　c. allow B to A　　d. stop B from A

文法解説　【時制】

【例（本文）】

(1) Rapid progress has been made in reducing deaths among children under age five.（現在完了形）
(2) An estimated 6.9 million children died before their fifth birthday, compared to around 12 million in 1990.（過去形）
(3) He calls this important progress.（現在形）
(4) Some 19,000 children are still dying every day from largely preventable causes.（現在進行形）

英語には「現在時制」「過去時制」「未来時制」の3つ時制があり、さらにそれぞれにはいくつかの形があります。

【時制の形と意味】

時制		形	意味
現在時制	現在形	動詞の原形と同じ 動詞の原形＋(e)s	① 現在の状態 ② 現在の反復動作 ③ 一般的事実や心理 ④ 確定した未来の予定
	現在進行形	am / is / are ＋ ing形	① 現在進行中の動作 ② 一定期間繰り返し行われている動作 ③ 未来の予定
	現在完了形	have / has ＋ 過去分詞形	① 完了・結果　　② 継続 ③ 経験
	現在完了進行形	have / has ＋ been ＋ ing形	① 動作の継続
過去時制	過去形	規則動詞：動詞の原形＋(e)d 不規則動詞	① 過去の状態　　② 過去の動作
	過去進行形	was / were ＋ ing形	① 過去のある時点での進行中の動作 ② 過去のある一定期間繰り返し行われていた動作 ③ 過去から見た未来の予定
	過去完了形	had ＋ 過去分詞形	過去のある時点での ① 完了・結果　　② 継続 ③ 経験　　　　　④ 大過去
	過去完了進行形	had ＋ been ＋ ing形	① 過去の動作の継続
未来時制	未来形	will〔be going to〕＋ 動詞の原形	① 単純未来　　② 意志未来
	未来進行形	will be ＋ ing形	① 未来のある時点での進行中の動作 ② 未来のある時点の予定の動作
	未来完了形	will have ＋ 過去分詞形	未来のある時点での ① 完了・結果　　② 継続 ③ 経験
	未来完了進行形	will have ＋ been ＋ ing形	① 未来のある時点までの動作の継続

※心理（like, love, know, want など）や知覚（see, hear など）、状態（be, remain, have, resemble など）を表す動詞は、原則として進行形になりません。

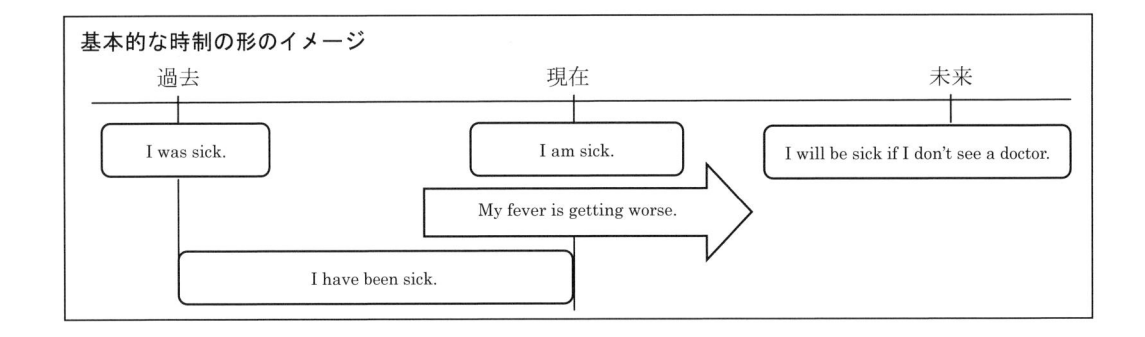

```
基本的な時制の形のイメージ
        過去              現在              未来
    ┌─────────┐      ┌─────────┐      ┌──────────────────────────┐
    │I was sick.│      │I am sick.│      │I will be sick if I don't │
    └─────────┘      └─────────┘      │see a doctor.             │
                                       └──────────────────────────┘
              My fever is getting worse.
         ┌──────────────────┐
         │I have been sick. │
         └──────────────────┘
```

文法問題　日本文を参考に、次の1～10の英文中の（　）内の動詞を適切な形にしましょう。

1. 現在、薬を服用していますか。
   (Be) you (take) any medication now?

2. もう同意書にサインをしましたか。
   (Have) you (sign) the consent form yet?
   ※ consent form：同意書

3. 昨日彼は頭痛を訴えてはいませんでした。
   He didn't (complain) of a headache yesterday.
   ※ complain of ～：（苦痛など）を訴える

4. 痛みが続くようならば、医者に診てもらってください。
   Go to see a doctor if the pain (persist).

5. 彼女の消化器系はその時回復のきざしを見せていた。
   Her digestive system (be) (show) signs of progress then.
   ※ digestive system：消化器（系）

6. 減量と適度な運動を心がければ、糖尿病になる危険性は低下するでしょう。
   Weight reduction and moderate exercise will (decrease) your risk of developing diabetes.
   ※ diabetes：糖尿病

7. 彼女は医者に自分の夫が前立腺がんで3年前に亡くなったことを語った。
   She told the doctor that her husband (have) (die) of prostate cancer three years before.
   ※ prostate cancer：前立腺がん

8. これまでに心臓発作を起こしたことがありますか。
   (Have) you (suffer) from a heart attack before?

9. たった4カ月の免疫療法で、腫瘍は劇的に縮小した。
   The tumor dramatically (shrink) with just four months of immunotherapy.
   ※ tumor：腫瘍　　immunotherapy：免疫療法

10. この病院の面会時間は午後1時から3時までです。
    This hospital's visiting hours (be) from one to three in the afternoon.

Chapter 14 世界の子どもたちの現状を知ろう！

英作文　次の日本文を英語になおしましょう。
1. 検査時間はおよそ10分です。（未来形を用いて）
2. （あなたの）血圧は上が126で下が90です。
3. 手術（operation）を受けたことはありますか。
4. 彼はサッカーの試合中に足を骨折した。
5. たばこを吸わなければ、気管支炎（bronchitis）はよくなるでしょう。

Let's think!

子どもがかかりやすい病気にはどのようなものがあるのか考えてみましょう。
　【例】rubella, mumps, chickenpox, etc.

Let's make a speech!

子どもがかかりやすい病気の原因、症状、治療法について、参考文献やインターネットなどを調べてまとめ、英語で3分間のスピーチをしてみましょう。

Column [コラム]　ミレニアム開発目標(Millennium Development Goals: MDGs)

　ミレニアム開発目標は、国連ミレニアム宣言（2000年9月の国連ミレニアム・サミットで採択）を基に掲げられた、2015年までに達成すべき8つの目標です。
目標1：極度の貧困と飢餓の撲滅　・1日1.25ドル未満で生活する人口の割合を半減させる
　　　　　　　　　　　　　　　　・飢餓に苦しむ人口の割合を半減させる
目標2：初等教育の完全普及の達成
　　　　　・すべての子どもが男女の区別なく初等教育の全課程を修了できるようにする
目標3：ジェンダー平等推進と女性の地位向上
　　　　　・すべての教育レベルにおける男女格差を解消する
目標4：乳幼児死亡率の削減　　・5歳未満児の死亡率を3分の1に削減する
目標5：妊産婦の健康の改善　　・妊産婦の死亡率を4分の1に削減する
目標6：HIV／エイズ、マラリア、その他の疾病の蔓延の防止
　　　　　・HIV／エイズの蔓延を阻止し、その後減少させる
目標7：環境の持続可能性確保
　　　　　・安全な飲料水と衛生施設を利用できない人口の割合を半減させる
目標8：開発のためのグローバルなパートナーシップの推進
　　　　　・民間部門と協力し、情報・通信分野の新技術による利益が得られるようにする

　ミレニアム開発目標の達成期限である2015年が迫る中、2015年以降の国際開発目標（ポストMDGs）の策定に向けた議論も始まっています。

Chapter 15　医師になるのはいばらの道

医師になるのは日本でも狭き門ですが、アメリカでも医師になる競争は激しいようです。日本とは違った教育システムを学んでください。

CD Track 16

So You Want to Make Your Mother Happy? Become a Doctor

Vocabulary Check（英文を読む前に意味を確認しましょう。）

- the Princeton Review：ザ・プリンストン・レビュー（大学入学試験対策や入学についての相談を業務とする民間企業） ▶ applicant：志願者
- the Medical College Admission Test：医科大学入学テスト（略称　MCAT）
- The Association of American Medical Colleges：米国医科大学協会 ▶ reasoning：論理的思考
- physical and biological sciences：自然科学と生物科学 ▶ do well：立派にやる、成功する
- representative：代表者 ▶ Public Health Service：米国公衆衛生局
- the F. Edward Hébert School of Medicine of the Uniformed Services University of the Health Sciences：軍人保健科学大学 F・エドワード・ハーバート医学部
- in return：その代わりに ▶ specialty：専門 ▶ intern：インターン（1年目の研修医）
- resident：レジデント（研修医） ▶ trainee：訓練を受けている人
- residency　医学部卒業後の専門医学実習

・自信のある人は英文をできるだけ速く読み、時間を計ってください。苦手な人はゆっくり読みましょう。

　It is not easy to become a doctor in the United States. The first step is getting into a medical college. More than one hundred twenty American schools offer study programs for people wanting to be doctors. People can get advice about medical schools from many resources. One of these is the Princeton Review. The publication provides information about colleges, study programs and jobs. The Princeton Review says competition to enter medical schools is strong. American medical schools have only about sixteen thousand openings for students. But more than two times this many seek entry. Many of those seeking to be admitted are women.

　Most people seeking admission contact more than one medical school. Some applicants contact many. An important part of the application usually is the Medical College Admission Test, or MCAT. The Association of American Medical Colleges provides the test by computer. It is offered in the United States and in other countries.

　The applicant is rated on reasoning, physical and biological sciences and an example of writing. Applicants for medical school need to do well on the MCAT. They also need a good record in their college studies.

　People who want to become doctors often study a lot of biology, chemistry or other science. Some students work for a year or two in a medical or research job before they attempt to enter medical school. A direct meeting, or interview, also is usually required for entrance to medical schools. This means talking with a school representative. The interviewer wants to know if the person understands the demands of life as a medical student and doctor in training. The interviewer wants to know about the person's goals for a life in medicine.

A medical education can cost a lot. One year at a private medical college can cost forty thousand dollars or more. The average cost at a public medical school is more than fifteen thousand dollars. Most students need loans to pay for medical school. Many finish their education heavily in debt. Some Americans become doctors by joining the United States Army, Navy, Air Force or Public Health Service. They attend the F. Edward Hébert School of Medicine of the Uniformed Services University of the Health Sciences in Bethesda, Maryland. These students attend without having to pay. In return, they spend seven years in government service. Doctors are among the highest paid people in the United States. Big-city doctors who work in specialties like eye care usually earn the most money. But some other doctors earn far less. That is especially true in poor communities.

Doctors-in-training in hospitals are known as interns or residents. They are usually called interns during their first year. After that, the name of the job is resident. The trainees treat patients guided by medical professors and other experts. All fifty states require at least one year of hospital work for doctors-in-training educated at medical schools in the United States. Graduates of study programs at most foreign medical schools may have to complete two or three years of residency, although there are exceptions.

(510 words)

(Voice of America, Special English, June 1, 2009)

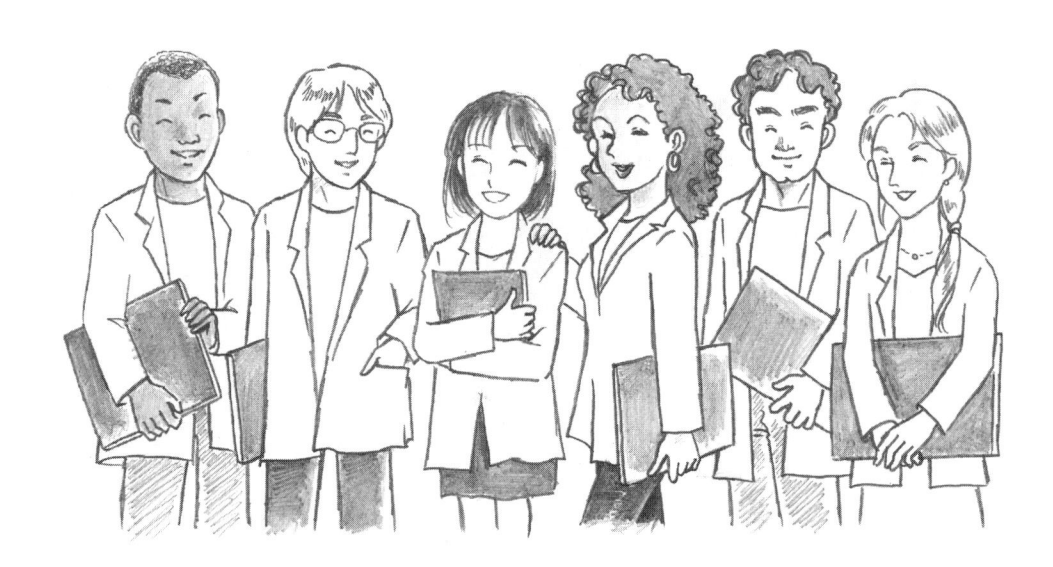

速読をした人は wpm を確認しましょう。

計算式：（あなたの wpm）＝ 510 /（かかった時間（分））　　　あなたの wpm：　　　　　wpm

(参考)
2.5分	204wpm	3分	170wpm	3.5分	146wpm
4分	128wpm	4.5分	113wpm	5分	102wpm
5.5分	93wpm	6分	85wpm		

内容把握問題　次の1～5の英文が、本文の内容と一致する場合はT、一致しない場合はFを（　）内に記入しましょう。

1. (　) Around 80 American schools offer study programs for people who want to become doctors.
2. (　) The Princeton Review doesn't say that the competition to enter medical schools is intense.
3. (　) Talking with a school representative is usually required for entrance to medical schools in the U.S.
4. (　) A medical education can cost a lot, but medical students can attend the F. Edward Hébert School of Medicine without paying tuition fees.
5. (　) Doctors in training are required to work at least two years in hospitals in the U.S.

上記の問題はいくつできましたか？　正解率をあなたの wpm の値にかけてみましょう。

計算式：（あなたの読解効率）＝（あなたの wpm）×（（正答数）/ 5）　　　あなたの読解効率：

語句問題　本文中に出てくる次の1～5の語句とほぼ同じ意味を表すものを a～d の中から1つ選びましょう。

1. offer
   a. publicize　　b. delete　　c. increase　　d. provide
2. publication
   a. book　　b. TV program　　c. school　　d. company
3. attempt
   a. study　　b. try　　c. fail　　d. succeed
4. expert
   a. generalist　　b. staff　　c. teacher　　d. specialist
5. complete
   a. escape　　b. finish　　c. skip　　d. purchase

文法解説【品詞】

「語」は、その意味や形態、文中での働きによって8つの品詞に分けられます。

① **名詞**　　人や物事の名を表す語
　【例】doctor, nurse, patient, lung, liver, brain, hospital, stethoscope, ventilator, ambulance など。

② **代名詞**　　名詞の代わりをする語
　【例】I, you, he, she, they, we, it など。

③ **形容詞**　　名詞・代名詞を限定・修飾する語
　【例】painful, infectious, intensive, allergic, intravenous, neonatal, surgical, critical, pregnant など。

④ **副詞**　　動詞・形容詞・他の副詞などを限定・修飾する語
　【例】immediately, chronically, terminally, suddenly, seldom, soon, very, unfortunately など。

⑤ **動詞**　　動作・状態を表す語
　【例】diagnose, bleed, breathe, resuscitate, admit, administer, sedate, push, deliver, treat など。

⑥ **前置詞**　　名詞・代名詞の前に置いて、形容詞句や副詞句をつくる語
　【例】at, in, on, from, to, for, along, across, into, over, under, above, below など。

⑦ **接続詞**　　語と語、句と句、節と節を結びつける語
　【例】and, but, or, when, because, if, though, while, since など。

⑧ **間投詞**　　さまざまな感情を表したり、よびかけたりする語
　【例】oh, ah, wow, oops, hi, hello など。

文法問題 次のA〜Eの英文の下線部の品詞（文中での働き）を答えましょう。

A. ①You should ②see a ③doctor ④about that ⑤cough.
B. I ⑥visited the doctor ⑦yesterday ⑧for a ⑨medical examination.
C. Peter and Carol ⑩work ⑪at the ⑫same trauma center.
D. ⑬If I had more time, I would ⑭learn ⑮another ⑯language.
E. "I ⑰am a ⑱nurse." "⑲Oh, ⑳really?"

英作文 次の日本文を英語になおしましょう。

1. ウェルビー医師（Dr. Welby）は彼の患者たちにとても人気がある。
2. 私は牛乳アレルギーだ（be allergic to）。
3. その女性は腹部を撃たれた（shot in the stomach）あと、出血多量で死亡した（bleed to death）。
4. 彼の娘は肝炎（hepatitis）であると診断された（be diagnosed with〔as〕）。
5. 彼女の母親は集中治療室（intensive care unit）へ入院させられた（be admitted to）。

Let's think!

アメリカと日本の医学教育の相違点について調べてみましょう。さらにアメリカと日本の医療保険制度の相違点についても調べてみましょう。〔参考：映画『シッコ』（*SiCKO*、マイケル・ムーア監督）〕そして、医療の世界でも日米に大きな相違点があることを認識しましょう。

Let's make a speech!

今まで診察を受けた日本人医師について思い出してみましょう。よかった点、よくなかった点をまとめ、日本の医師像について3分間のスピーチをしてみましょう。

> **Column** [コラム]
>
> ## 「アメリカの医学教育」
>
> 　米国で医師になるためには、4年制大学を卒業後、さらに医学校において4年間の医学教育を受けなくてはなりません。医学校を卒業すると医学士（M. D.）となりますが、一人前の医師になるためには、レジデンシー（residency）とよばれる臨床研修を受ける必要があり、臨床研修を受ける研修医はレジデント（resident）、とくに1年目の研修医はインターン（intern）とよばれます。レジデンシーの期間は専門分野によって異なります。内科で2年目、外科で2年目・3年目の研修医はジュニア・レジデント（junior resident）、内科で3年目、外科で4年目・5年目の研修医はシニア・レジデント（senior resident）とよばれます。米国の過酷な研修医な生活を描いたものに *Rotations: The 12 Months of Intern Life*（日本語版は『アメリカ新人研修医の挑戦　最高で最低で最悪の12ヵ月』（西村書店））や *The Making of a Surgeon in the 21st Century*（日本語版は『外科研修医　熱き混沌(カオス)』（医歯薬出版））があります。

解答

Answer

Chapter 1

A.

内容把握問題
1. T　　2. F　　3. T　　4. T　　5. F

語句問題
1. b　　2. b　　3. d　　4. a　　5. d

B.

内容把握問題
1. F　　2. F　　3. F　　4. T　　5. F

語句問題
1. b　　2. b　　3. d　　4. d　　5. c

文法問題
1. 3　　2. 5　　3. 1　　4. 1　　5. 3
6. 4　　7. 2　　8. 5　　9. 3　　10. 2

英作文
1. The patient cannot walk without crutches.
2. I feel better〔good〕today.
3. I have a stomachache.
4. He lent me a walking stick.
5. I found my doctor (in charge) honest.

Chapter 2

内容把握問題
1. F　　2. F　　3. T　　4. T　　5. T

語句問題
1. a　　2. b　　3. b　　4. c　　5. d

文法問題　A　1. 単文　2. 複文　3. 重文　4. 単文　5. 複文

B　1. does, not, produce　　2. Were, or
3. How, long, do, have　　4. Don't　　5. How

英作文
1. I have a bad〔terrible〕cough.
2. How is your appetite?
3. Take this medicine when you have a fever.
4. Did you wash your hands before the meal?
5. It is important to blow your nose when you have a cold.

Chapter 3

内容把握問題 1. F   2. T   3. F   4. T   5. T
語句問題   1. b   2. a   3. b   4. d   5. d
文法問題   1. a   2. b   3. d   4. a   5. d
                6. a   7. d   8. c   9. b   10. a

英作文
1. Doctors must [should] listen to what patients say.
2. The doctor who treated her said she would recover soon.
3. Lungs are organs that are used for breathing.
4. A nurse [Nurses] encouraged the son whose father was in a coma.
5. Please show me the ankle you sprained yesterday.

Chapter 4

内容把握問題 1. F   2. F   3. T   4. T   5. T
語句問題   1. c   2. b   3. a   4. c   5. b
文法問題   1. why   2. when   3. why   4. where   5. how
                6. where   7. why   8. where   9. when   10. how

英作文
1. This is how I studied medicine.
2. We moved to Tokyo, where we opened a clinic.
3. I sometimes wonder why I became a nurse.
4. There are many [a lot of] reasons (why) people develop heart disease.
5. This is the medical center where my father works.

Chapter 5

内容把握問題 1. F   2. F   3. T   4. F   5. T
語句問題   1. a   2. d   3. d   4. b   5. b
文法問題
1. Walking down the street, I met Dr. Kitano.
2. All things being equal, the simplest explanation is the best.
3. Being a vegetarian, the patient doesn't eat any kind of meat.
4. I fell down, striking my head against the door.
5. She entered the consulting room, accompanied by her mother.
6. Being badly injured, she couldn't walk.
7. Asked some questions by his proffessor, the student was not able to answer.
8. Despite having a fever, she took the entrance examination.
9. It being a fine day, we decided to take the patient for a walk.
10. Having received their medical check, the astronauts boarded their spacecraft.

英作文
1. Being tired, I went to bed earlier last night.
2. Having a cold, I went to see [saw] a doctor yesterday.
3. Studying hard, the student passed the national exam for medical practitioners.
4. Not knowing what to do, she asked a [the] nurse for advice.
5. Looking at her doctor (in charge), she smiled.

Chapter 6

内容把握問題
1. T   2. F   3. T   4. F   5. T

語句問題
1. d   2. a   3. c   4. b   5. a

文法問題
1. exposed   2. using   3. contained   4. making
5. suffering   6. left   7. sleeping   8. exhausted
9. recovering   10. prolonged

英作文
1. The number of old people living alone has been increasing.
2. People suffering from life-threatening diseases are exposed to severe stress.
3. The two workers transported by ambulance after the explosion were died on arrival [when they arrived at the hospital].
4. The medical team selected by the goverment included clinical psychologists and psychiatrists.
5. There are data showing [Some data shows] that people transported by air ambulance have a high survival rate.

Chapter 7

内容把握問題
1. F   2. T   3. F   4. T   5. T

語句問題
1. a   2. c   3. a   4. a   5. b

文法問題
1. C   2. B   3. C   4. B   5. C
6. C   7. A   8. A   9. B   10. A

英作文
1. I would like to make an appointment with a doctor [to see a doctor].
2. It is necessary for you to see a doctor.
3. Be careful not to catch a cold.
4. The patient is difficult to please.
5. The doctor advised her to take a complete rest.

Chapter 8

内容把握問題
1. F   2. T   3. F   4. T   5. T

語句問題
1. b   2. b   3. d   4. a   5. d

文法問題
A   1. developing   2. taking   3. visualizing
    4. Reading   5. enhancing
B   1. On, hearing   2. his [him], getting   3. use, worrying
    4. like, eating   5. without saying

英作文
1. I stopped smoking two years ago.
2. The first step is getting into (entering) a medical college.
3. The patient is looking forward to seeing his [her] family.
4. There is no telling what will happen tomorrow.
5. I remember seeing the patient once.

Chapter 9

内容把握問題 1. F 2. F 3. F 4. T 5. T
語句問題 1. b 2. d 3. b 4. d 5. a
文法問題 A
1. The doctor is respected by every patient.
2. I was shown the way to the waiting room by the nurse.
   The way to the waiting room was shown to me by the nurse.
3. The medicine is being taken by him.
4. He was given an injection by the doctor.
   An injection was given to him by the doctor.
5. Thousands of "laughter clubs" have been inspired by his movement.
6. Laughter sessions are held by Kataria.
7. Laughter yoga will help her.
8. The doctor makes many patients happy.
9. They had to persuade him to laugh.
10. The bite of an infected mosquito causes malaria.

英作文
1. He was saved by his wife's smile.
2. My mother was treated by three doctors.
3. A tired soul is healed by music.
4. Aromatherapy is used to reduce patients' tension.
5. My favorite herbal tea is sold at convenience stores.

Chapter 10

内容把握問題 1. F 2. T 3. T 4. F 5. T
語句問題 1. b 2. d 3. a 4. d 5. c
文法問題
1. didn't, have   2. had, not, seen [met]   3. got, hit
4. had, drunk, not, be   5. had, been   6. explained
7. were   8. had, had   9. were   10. could, leave

英作文
1. I wish I were a doctor.
2. The patient behaves as if he [she] were a child.
3. If iPS cells had been discovered earlier, he could have been saved.
4. If the government approved the clinical test, the researchers could start the study soon.
5. If the Japanese government had supported the young researcher, he could have received the Nobel Prize.

Chapter 11

内容把握問題
1. F 2. T 3. F 4. T 5. T

語句問題
1. a 2. b 3. d 4. a 5. c

文法問題
1. What   2. how   3. what   4. whether
5. What〔Which〕   6. How many   7. What   8. Where
9. What   10. whose

英作文
1. When was the sale of nonprescription drugs over the Internet allowed?
2. Who is responsibe for online sales of drugs?
3. Do you know when the law went into force?
4. Please tell me where the drug is sold.
5. I don't know how I can〔how to〕get information on the drug.

Chapter 12

内容把握問題
1. F 2. T 3. F 4. T 5. F

語句問題
1. a 2. b 3. d 4. a 5. c

文法問題
1. neither   2. nor   3. no   4. little
5. no   6. not   7. few   8. hardly
9. no   10. fail to eradicate

英作文
1. There is little doubt that the fetus has a chromosomal abnormality.
2. An amniotic fluid check is seldom used in the hospital.
3. The hospital had neither full-time obstetricians nor pediatricians.
4. Not all pregnant women take a prenatal blood test.
5. No mention was made of the new prenatal diagnosis.

Chapter 13

内容把握問題
1. F 2. T 3. T 4. F 5. F

語句問題
1. a 2. d 3. b 4. c 5. a

文法問題
1. Keep   2. fill   3. contact   4. take
5. Let, explain   6. Go, turn   7. get〔take〕   8. Don't, drive
9. lie   10. Don't, eat〔drink〕, drink〔eat〕

英作文
1. Take a deep breath and hold it.
2. Take this medicine〔drug〕twice a day.
3. Take care of yourself.
4. Let me take your blood pressure.
5. Don't worry.

Chapter 14

内容把握問題
1. F　　2. T　　3. T　　4. T　　5. F

語句問題
1. b　　2. d　　3. b　　4. c　　5. a

文法問題
1. Are, taking　　2. Have, signed　　3. complain
4. persists　　5. was, showing　　6. decrease
7. had, died　　8. Have, suffered　　9. shrank　　10. are

英作文
1. The examination will take about 10 minutes.
2. Your blood pressure is 126 over 90.
3. Have you (ever) had any operations [undergone surgery]?
4. He broke a bone in his leg [broke his leg] while (he was) playing soccer.
5. If you don't smoke [Unless you smoke], your bronchitis will get better.

Chapter 15

内容把握問題
1. F　　2. F　　3. T　　4. T　　5. F

語句問題
1. d　　2. a　　3. b　　4. d　　5. b

文法問題
①代名詞　　②動詞　　③名詞　　④前置詞
⑤名詞　　⑥動詞　　⑦副詞　　⑧前置詞
⑨形容詞　　⑩動詞　　⑪前置詞　　⑫形容詞
⑬接続詞　　⑭動詞　　⑮形容詞　　⑯名詞
⑰動詞　　⑱名詞　　⑲間投詞　　⑳副詞

英作文
1. Dr. Welby is very popular with [among] his patients.
2. I'm allergic to (cow's) milk.
3. The woman bled to death after being shot [she was shot] in the stomach.
4. His daughter was diagnosed with [as] hepatitis.
5. Her mother was admitted [was made to admit] to the intensive care unit.

編著者紹介

川越　栄子
かわごえ　えいこ

神戸女学院大学大学院文学研究科修士課程修了
神戸女学院大学共通英語教育研究センター教授・センター長、
大阪大学非常勤講師等を経て、
現在、滋慶医療科学大学教授、神戸大学医学部医学科・保健学科非常勤講師

NDC 490　　110p　　26cm

ニュースで読む医療英語　CD付き
よ　　いりょうえいご　　つ

2014 年 8 月 28 日　第 1 刷発行
2025 年 1 月 16 日　第 8 刷発行

編著者	川越栄子（かわごええいこ）
発行者	篠木和久
発行所	株式会社　講談社　KODANSHA
	〒112-8001　東京都文京区音羽 2-12-21
	販　売　(03) 5395-5817
	業　務　(03) 5395-3615
編集	株式会社　講談社サイエンティフィク
	代表　堀越俊一
	〒162-0825　東京都新宿区神楽坂 2-14　ノービィビル
	編　集　(03) 3235-3701
印刷所	株式会社ＫＰＳプロダクツ
製本所	株式会社国宝社

落丁本・乱丁本は，購入書店名を明記のうえ，講談社業務宛にお送りください．送料小社負担にてお取替えいたします．なお，この本の内容についてのお問い合わせは，講談社サイエンティフィク宛にお願いいたします．価格はカバーに表示してあります．

© Eiko Kawagoe, 2014

本書のコピー，スキャン，デジタル化等の無断複製は著作権法上での例外を除き禁じられています．本書を代行業者等の第三者に依頼してスキャンやデジタル化することはたとえ個人や家庭内の利用でも著作権法違反です．

Printed in Japan

ISBN978-4-06-156310-0

やさしい英語ニュースで学ぶ 現代社会と健康
田中 芳文・編著
B5・110頁・定価2,640円（税込）
健康・医療・生活のニュースでトレーニングする英語教科書。一般向け記事なので、現代社会とのつながりを意識しながらスラスラ読める。
ISBN 978-4-06-155633-1

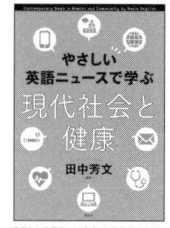

英文ニュースで学ぶ 健康とライフスタイル
田中 芳文・編著
B5・112頁・定価2,860円（税込）
医療や健康の話題を扱ったニュース記事で英語リーディング能力をレベルアップ！ 一般人向けの記事だから、出てくる用語は一般常識レベルで、文章も読みやすい。看護系や健康栄養系の学生のための新しい英語トレーニング！
ISBN978-4-06-155629-4

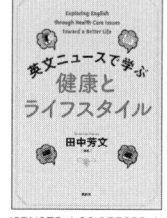

ニュースで読む医療英語
CD付き
川越 栄子・編著
森 茂／田中 芳文／名木田 恵理子／大下 晴美・著
B5・112頁・定価3,080円（税込）
医療・看護のためのやさしい英語テキスト。一般向けのわかりやすい医療ニュースを題材に、入門レベルの読者でもすらすら読める。ネイティブ読み上げCD付きでリスニングもバッチリ！
ISBN978-4-06-156310-0

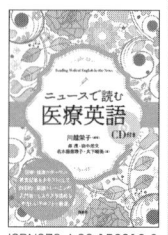

やさしい栄養英語
田中 芳文・編著
中里 菜穂子／松浦 加寿子・著
B5・64頁・定価1,980円（税込）
英語の栄養学読み物を題材にした教科書。一般向けの読み物だから、簡単な英文でスラスラ読める。栄養学の基礎も身について一石二鳥！
用語説明も充実しているので、辞書をひく必要なし。英文の長さや問題の量、全体のページ数に至るまで、スッキリ学べる手ごろな分量。
ISBN 978-4-06-513414-6

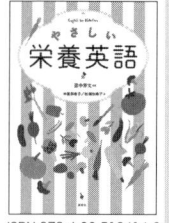

はじめての栄養英語
えっ、Dietって、やせるって意味じゃないの？
栄養士の私はDietitianなんだ！
美味しく学べる英語のスキル
清水 雅子・著
B5・112頁・定価1,980円（税込）
やさしい英文で初学者でも栄養英語に親しめるよう工夫されたテキスト。栄養素、代謝、解剖生理、消化吸収、食品添加物、食物アレルギーなどを、やさしく短い英文でとりあげた。
ISBN978-4-06-155613-3

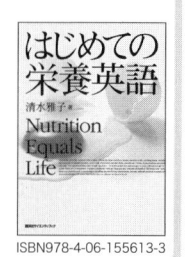

はじめての臨床栄養英語
清水 雅子／J. パトリック・バロン・著
B5・128頁・定価2,530円（税込）
栄養管理を必要とする疾患を中心に、平易な英文で、組織・器官の名称、病気の概要、診断基準、食事療法、薬物療法を学ぶ、これまでにない教科書。病院臨地実習やゼミで必須となる基本英語を集約。大学院受験にも役立つ1冊。
ISBN978-4-06-155621-8

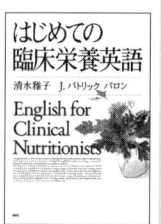

Let's Study English!
Health and Nutrition
英語で読む健康と栄養
横尾 信男・編著
A5・96頁・定価1,650円（税込）
栄養系学生のための教養課程英語テキスト。健康な食生活に必要な知識（栄養素やその摂取法、病気にならない食生活・エクササイズ、酒やタバコの害、食中毒、ストレス解消など）を幅広く学べるように編集。
ISBN978-4-06-153951-8

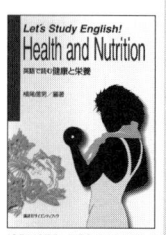

耳から学ぶ 楽しいナース英語
CD付き
中西 睦子・監修 野口 ジュディー／川越 栄子／仁平 雅子・著
B5・112頁・定価3,740円（税込）
CDを聞きながら学ぶ看護英語の決定版。国際化時代の医療現場では英語は不可欠の時代、聞きとれること話せることは必要要素。「どうかしましたか」「どのように痛みますか」こんな会話が話せるようになる1冊。
ISBN978-4-06-153672-2

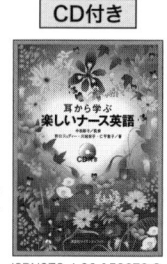

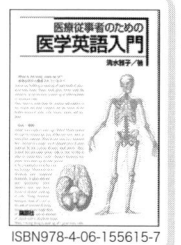

医療従事者のための 医学英語入門
清水 雅子・著
A5・216頁・定価2,750円（税込）
人体組織、器官を中心に基礎医学をコンパクトに収載した1991年刊の好評テキスト『医療技術者のための医学英語入門』が新版となって登場。図版も追加され、さらに使いやすくなった。
ISBN978-4-06-155615-7

英語で学ぶプライマリーケア
西牟田 祐美子・編著
B5・112頁・定価2,200円（税込）
読んで楽しい看護学生向けテキスト。カラー4コマ漫画を手始めに、看護現場の様子を英語で学ぶことができる。リーディング、文法、演習問題も掲載。リスニング教材をホームページからダウンロード可能。
ISBN978-4-06-520090-2

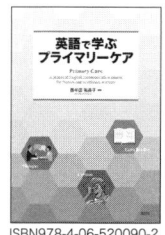

講談社サイエンティフィク　https://www.kspub.co.jp/

※表示価格は消費税(10%)が加算されています。

2025年1月現在